MILITARY PSYCHIATRY

OTHER BOOKS BY RICHARD A. GABRIEL

Military Incompetence: Why the US Military Doesn't Win

Operation Peace for Galilee: The Israeli-PLO War in Lebanon

The Antagonists: A Comparative Combat Assessment of the Soviet and American Soldier

The Mind of the Soviet Fighting Man

To Serve With Honor: A Treatise on Military Ethics and the Way of the Soldier

Fighting Armies: NATO and the Warsaw Pact

Fighting Armies: Antagonists of the Middle East

Fighting Armies: Third World Armies

The New Red Legions: An Attitudinal Portrait of the Soviet Soldier

The New Red Legions: A Survey Data Sourcebook

Crisis in Command: Mismanagement in the US Army

Managers and Gladiators: Directions of Change In the US Army

Ethnic Groups in America

Program Evaluation: A Social Science Approach

The Ethnic Factor in the Urban Polity

The Environment: Critical Factors in Strategy Development

Soviet Military Psychiatry: The Theory and Practice of Coping with Battle Stress

MILITARY PSYCHIATRY

A COMPARATIVE PERSPECTIVE

EDITED BY
Richard A. Gabriel

CONTRIBUTIONS IN MILITARY STUDIES,
NUMBER 57

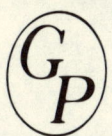

GREENWOOD PRESS
NEW YORK · WESTPORT, CONNECTICUT · LONDON

Library of Congress Cataloging-in-Publication Data

Military psychiatry.

(Contributions in military studies, ISSN 0883-6884 ; no. 57)
Bibliography: p.
Includes index.
1. Psychiatry, Military.   I. Gabriel, Richard A.
II. Series.
UH629.M55   1986   616.85′212   86-12107
ISBN 0-313-25491-5 (lib. bdg. : alk. paper)

Copyright © 1986 by Richard Gabriel

All rights reserved. No portion of this book may be reproduced, by any process or technique, without the express written consent of the publisher.

Library of Congress Catalog Card Number: 86-12107
ISBN: 0-313-25491-5
ISSN: 0883-6884

First published in 1986

Greenwood Press, Inc.
88 Post Road West, Westport, Connecticut 06881

Printed in the United States of America

The paper used in this book complies with the Permanent Paper Standard issued by the National Information Standards Organization (Z39.48-1984).

10 9 8 7 6 5 4 3 2 1

For Pat and Bill Lake . . .
And for Noah. Welcome to the
world, kid . . . Protect yourself at
all times!

Contents

TABLES ix
FIGURES xi

Introduction 1
Richard A. Gabriel

1. The Human Dimension of Battle and Combat Breakdown 7
   David Marlowe

2. American Military Psychiatry 25
   Lawrence Ingraham and Frederick Manning

3. Soviet Military Psychiatry 67
   Richard A. Gabriel

4. Military Psychiatry in the German Army 119
   Robert Schneider

5. Military Psychiatry in the Israeli Defense Force 147
   Gregory Lucas Belenky

6. Future Directions of Military Psychiatry 181
   Franklin D. Jones

BIBLIOGRAPHIC ESSAY   205

INDEX   209

CONTRIBUTORS   213

Tables

2.1	Men Rejected for Military Service and Enlisted Men Separated from the Army for Emotional or Mental Reasons, World War I and World War II	35
3.1	Drugs Used by Soviet Military Psychiatrists in Treatment of Neurosis and Psychosis	105
3.2	Symptom Indicators Used by Soviet Military Psychiatrists to Diagnose Battle Neurosis and Psychosis	107
3.3	Common Terms Used in Western Military Psychiatry That Are Not Used by Soviet Military Psychiatrists	107
5.1	Physical Casualties in Israeli Forces in Lebanon, June–December 1982	157
5.2	Incidence of Psychiatric Casualties (Battle-Shock and Mixed Syndromes) in Israeli Forces in Lebanon, June–December 1982	157
5.3	Symptoms Reported by Psychiatric Casualties in Israeli Forces in Lebanon, June–September 1982	160
5.4	Psychiatric Symptom Clusters in Different Wars, Both U.S. and Israeli	161

5.5	Results of Treatment of Psychiatric Casualties in Israeli Forces in Lebanon, June–September 1982	163
5.6	Factors Correlated with Return to Duty Following Psychiatric Breakdown in Israeli Forces in Lebanon, June–September 1982	166
5.7	Combat Fitness Retraining Unit (CFRU), Third Echelon of Treatment of Battle-Shock Casualties in Israeli Forces in Lebanon, June–September 1982	167
5.8	Recurrence of Battle-Shock in Israeli Forces in Lebanon, June–September 1982	169
5.9	Battle Stress as a Predictor of Battle-Shock, Israeli Forces in Lebanon, June–September 1982	170
5.10	Ratio of Battle-Shock to Wounded by Age in Israeli Forces in Lebanon, June–September 1982	172
5.11	Correlations Between Morale and Other Variables in Israeli Forces, May 1981	173
6.1	Symptom Clusters in Various Wars	186
6.2	Factors and Characteristics of Nostalgic Casualties	189
6.3	Characteristics of High-Intensity Warfare	193
6.4	Negation of Principles of Forward Treatment	193
6.5	Principles of Combat Psychiatry in High-Intensity Warfare	196

Figures

2.1 Discharge Rates of Enlisted Men for Neuropsychiatric Conditions, U.S. Army, by Year and Month, 1942–1945   36

2.2 Admission Rates for Neuropsychiatric Disorders, U.S. Army, by Year and Month, 1942–1945   37

4.1 Diagnoses of Patients Admitted to the Ensen Military Hospital   138

MILITARY PSYCHIATRY

Introduction

RICHARD A. GABRIEL

One of the most important elements in the equation of an army's combat effectiveness is how well soldiers stand up to the horrors of battle. In the end, all war is a series of small wars comprised of hundreds of small-unit engagements in which the ability of human beings to endure is crucial to the unit's success or failure. In an age when military thinkers stress the technology of war—the killing power of modern weaponry—it is often forgotten that the effectiveness of any weapon, no matter how destructive, ultimately depends on the ability of a single human being or small groups of human beings to operate it. Technology, no matter how destructive, will never obscure the role of the human element in achieving success on the field of battle.

The problem is that human beings are very fragile. No matter how well trained the soldier is, no matter how cohesive his units, no matter how good and technically proficient his leaders are, men in battle will succumb to the stresses and strains placed on them by their destructive environment. The experience of military history amply demonstrates that no one is immune to battle stress. Given enough combat over time, every soldier will eventually break down and cease to function.

The only question which military planners can realistically address in this regard is how to prevent the rates of combat stress breakdown from overwhelming an army's combat abilities. While strong, cohesive, disciplined, and well-led units can prevent rapid collapse or can delay somewhat the amount of time required for soldiers to become debilitated, the real challenge for military psychiatry is how to treat those who have already broken under stress and how quickly they can be returned to the battle. All other concerns are secondary.

The problem of manpower loss from psychiatric debilitation is fast reaching crisis proportions. As war becomes more destructive and the battlefield more lethal with the advent of each new generation of weapons, the number of men lost to the fighting effort as a result of mental collapse could materially reduce the combat power of fighting forces and, in some instances, overwhelm it altogether. In World War II, for example, American fighting forces lost 504,000 men from the fighting effort because of psychiatric collapse. That number would man fifty combat divisions! When measured against the stress and lethality of the contemporary battlefield, World War II battles pale in comparison. Thus, in the 1973 Arab-Israeli War, almost a third of all Israeli casualties were due to psychiatric causes. The same seems to have been true among the opposing Egyptian forces. In the 1982 incursion into Lebanon, Israeli psychiatric casualties were twice as high as the number of dead and accounted for about 27 percent of the total number of wounded casualties. Projections for future, purely conventional war scenarios involving a clash between Soviet and NATO forces in Central Europe suggest that the number of psychiatric casualties could reach between 40 and 50 percent of total casualties. In a scenario in which "limited" nuclear weapons would be used in Central Europe, the number of psychiatric casualties could reasonably be expected to increase even more. The problem of psychiatric breakdown in battle is thus becoming one of central importance for any military force that can expect to see battle in the near future.

Given the importance of preventing and treating combat stress casualties and the large amount of experience armies have had with the problem since at least 1905, by now armies should have developed relatively successful strategies for dealing with the problem. And to some extent this has been the case. All modern armies have established some plans, doctrines, and medical assets devoted to dealing with the problem. Yet, the field of military psychiatry is still very much a developing discipline in terms of definitively ascertaining which mechanisms work best. Although concerned military planners in every army are making some effort to study the experiences of other armies in this area, their results have been less than systematic and complete.

The doctrines and practices of each army are far more the result of its own battle experiences and the quality and direction of the broader field of psychiatry within its own country than of any systematic attempt to study and incorporate information available through military history or the experiences of other armies. That is why we have no comprehensive written history of military psychiatry that addresses the development of the discipline cross culturally. That is also why there are no books that offer a comparative in-depth treatment of the subject against the background of historical experience. Although a definitive history of military psychiatry in the West remains to be written, this book offers what we believe to be the first cross-cultural examination of military psychiatry as it has developed and is practiced by four major armies, the U.S., Soviet, German, and Israeli.

This work begins with a chapter on the human dimension of combat. Without an understanding of the role of the human psyche in dealing with the stress imposed on it by armed combat, no further progress is possible. In order to manage the problem of military effectiveness, military planners must first come to grips with the limitations of the mind which are imposed by its very fragility. At a near point in the future, if, indeed, we have not already reached it, war may become obsolete. That is, the practice of warfare may become impossible for the human being to perform. The limits of warfare are already clear, and chief among them is the ability of human beings to remain sane and functional amid the storm of horror that battle necessarily entails.

The next four chapters offer a detailed examination of the historical development and effectiveness of military psychiatry in four major armies. Not incidentally, these four armies appear to have the most developed and detailed doctrines and practices for dealing with psychiatric breakdown under fire. No doubt this reflects the fact that these are the most combat-experienced forces in the world. Apparently, in the field of military psychiatry, necessity is once again the mother of invention.

The work concludes with a chapter on the future directions of military psychiatry and on the question of whether any doctrine of preventing battle stress has any realistic chance of succeeding. Past approaches to the problem of stress casualties would likely no longer function except in low-intensity conflicts. Just where that leaves the individual soldier, to say nothing of the military planner, is a question whose implications stagger the imagination.

In analyzing the experiences of the four armies in the field of military psychiatry, the persistence of stress reactions is remarkable almost regardless of what military psychiatrists attempt to do about them. One can but marvel at the inventiveness of the human psyche in its efforts to escape its surrounding horror by generating all kinds of symptoms and behavioral conditions. There seems to be a clear connection between those symptoms which the soldier and psychiatric diagnosticians on the battlefield have been trained to recognize as "legitimate" reasons for removing the soldier from battle and the precise symptoms which soldiers manifest when subjected to battle stress. And there is no reason to believe that the inventiveness of the human psyche in this area has been exhausted. New conditions of stress will almost certainly generate new symptoms. The circle is as complete as it is vicious.

All of this raises the question of whether or not military psychiatrists may be wasting their time. If one believes that defining and recognizing certain symptoms as legitimate enough to remove the soldier from combat will result in the generating of these symptoms—which in turn, means that psychiatric cases will almost always tax the medical service structure—why not, then, enforce a harsh set of diagnostic criteria—as does the Soviet Army and did the German Army—and force the soldier to return to the fighting at gunpoint if necessary? After all, that is precisely what the Soviet and American armies intend to do with those soldiers who receive a fatal dose of radiation in the event of nuclear warfare. To be sure, these soldiers will eventually die—perhaps within a matter of four to five days. But why not, as the argument goes, get a few more days of combat power out of them?

The argument against using inflexible diagnostic categories is that cumulative stress will eventually manifest itself in some way regardless of what is done. Thus, if one does not treat acute anxiety, it will show up sooner or later in such things as self-inflicted wounds, higher numbers of accidental injuries, frostbite, incapacitating headaches, AWOL, and even the contracting of venereal disease. Granted that such expectations are correct, it is still unclear whether the time required for such manifestations to occur would not be longer than the time lost to treating the psychiatric casualty in the first place. It is also unclear whether it would not be easier to treat the physical debilitation—frostbite, venereal disease, and so on—than to treat the psychiatric conditions which military psychiatry currently addresses. Finally, success in treating physical conditons may be more rapid than in treating the underlying psychiatric condition. In treating physical injuries the soldier obtains much of the same treatment—rest, food, sleep, respite from battle—that he would obtain from becoming a purely psychiatric casualty. In short, strict diagnostic criteria will not eliminate psychiatric casualties, but they might make treatment easier while at the same time allowing the psychiatrically stressed soldier to function longer in the battlezone.

Although this debate will not likely reach an easy or rapid conclusion—indeed, the debate along these lines has hardly begun in earnest—the partial evidence found in military history suggests that something may be gained from pursuing it. In World War I, for example, almost all major combatants used a harsh diagnostic definition of what constituted a legitimate psychiatric casualty. In general, a soldier manifesting psychiatric symptoms had first to be found to be suffering from some organic cause of the symptom before he was granted relief from duty. Thus, psychiatric debilitation was attributed to such things as shell shock, microbleeding in the brain, and the commotion wrought on nerve pathways of the brain. Interestingly, most armies in that war suffered about the same level of manpower loss for psychiatric reasons—between six to nine men per thousand casualties, which is a comparatively low rate.

By World War II, some combatants had accepted more lenient diagnostic definitions for recognizing and treating psychiatric casualties, moving beyond purely organic causes to purely emotional and psychogenic causes. Other former World War I combatants retained their harsh organic defintions; comparing the performance of these two sets of combatants in World War II is very illuminating.

In World War I the American Army, utilizing strict diagnostic categories, suffered a psychiatric casualty rate of about nine men per thousand. In World War II, after it had adopted a more relaxed diagnostic system, the rate went up to thirty-six men per thousand, a rate four times higher. The Germans and Russians in World War I, who also suffered a rate of about nine per thousand, retained their harsh diagnostic definitions in World War II and both armies kept the rate of nine per thousand. By any standard, the manpower loss to psychiatric collapse was much lower in those armies that had not abandoned exacting diagnostic definitions. If it is true that the German and Soviet armies suffered large numbers of collateral psychiatric casualties—those soldiers whose psychiatric symptoms manifested themselves in more direct physical symptoms such as accidents, disease, and frostbite—the rates of occurrence of these types of casualties did not seem sufficient to weaken their battle performance.

None of this is to suggest that armies can dispense with military psychiatry. What it does suggest is that in an era of high-intensity warfare of greatly increased lethality some thought might be given to redefining the role, doctrine, and practices of military psychiatry in the battlezone to accommodate devastating realities. The sad truth is that soldiers have always been dispensable to some extent in war. Certainly, loss rates are somewhat predictable for certain kinds of operations. Perhaps we have reached a point where the cruel reality is that soldiers who suffer psychiatric difficulties are somewhat more dispensable than others. This proposition is especially cruel in view of the evidence that all men—regardless of personality traits—are at risk of mental collapse in the environment of modern war.

In the end, of course, there is no answer; there are only victims. The tragic realities of past wars have grown exponentially more tragic as nations face the prospect of future wars. The human material of warfare has not changed, nor is it likely to. The men who stood at Meggido or Cannae or Waterloo were no different from those who will be asked to stand on future battlefields. They will have the same hopes and the same fears, and all too many will suffer the same fate. What has changed, of course, is the nature, tempo, and lethality of war. Whereas in the past weaponry was molded to the human capacity to use it, today the human capacity must be molded to deal with the weaponry. It is by no means certain that the task is possible. Indeed, it may be impossible . . . and that simple fact could change everything.

1
The Human Dimension of Battle and Combat Breakdown

DAVID MARLOWE

The ultimate limiting factor for the maintenance and endurance of organized and competent forces on the battlefield is the human being. The contemporary soldier's combat environment is the most stressful, threatening, and alien to which any human being could be subject. Each man committed to battle is the locus of two sets of contending forces: those that would either physically or psychologically destroy him as a functional and capable combatant, and those that would maintain him.

The power of the battlefield to break men can never be overstated. As the intensity, lethality, and duration of time in which troops are engaged in exchanging direct and indirect fire with the enemy increases, the potentiality for individual breakdown and unit disruption also increases. History is our guide and is a compelling schoolmaster; and it is to history, particularly the history of World War II and the 1973 Arab-Israeli War that we must look for guidance to the worst case conventional wars of the future.

Although many of the principles underlying World War II were much the same for the Korean and Vietnam wars, the last two wars were

The views of the author do not purport to reflect the positions of the department of the army or the department of defense (Para 4-3, AR-360-5).

aberrant in the sense that the soldier's future was as much controlled by the calendar (Date of Expected Return from Overseas [DEROS]) as by the outcome of combat with the enemy. The Vietnam War was particularly variant in that the enemy lacked significant capacity in weapons of indirect fire, thus providing a battlefield ecology that was substantively different from both the past and the anticipated future. Much higher proportions of combat casualties in Vietnam were due to small arms and booby traps, as opposed to the greater proportion of artillery-inflicted wounds and deaths in World War II and in Korea. (Appel and Beebe, 1946; Musser and Stengers, 1972).

Thus, whereas the Vietnam conflict was no less stressful or deadly to the infantry platoon engaged in a desperate firefight with the enemy, such actions had neither the scale, the intensity, nor the duration of high-intensity main force battles between essentially equipotent forces utilizing massive resources for indirect fire. Nor did men see themselves as committed to the end of battle, as they of necessity would in any Central European scenario.

The capacity of severe and sustained combat to break men is great and can take many forms. The most readily assessable of these forms is that which is usually denoted as the combat psychiatric casualty—the individual suffering from "combat reaction" or "battle or combat fatigue." The proximate causes of such breakdowns are well known and have been described by many authorities:

The key to understanding of the psychiatric problem is the simple fact that the danger of being killed or maimed imposes a strain so great that it causes men to break down. One look at the shrunken apathetic faces of psychiatric cases as they come stumbling into the medical station, sobbing, trembling referring shudderingly to "them shells" and to buddies mutilated or dead is enough to convince most observers of this fact. There is no such thing as "getting used to combat." Each man "up there" knew that at any moment he might be killed, a fact kept constantly before his mind by the sight of dead and mutilated buddies around him. Each moment of combat imposes a strain so great that men will break down in direct relation to the intensity and duration of their exposure. Thus psychiatric casualties are as inevitable as gunshot and shrapnel wounds in warfare (Appel and Beebe, 1946, p. 84).

Who were these men? Almost all studies from World War II and Korea demonstrate that there were no special psychiatric predispositions to break down in battle. Men with histories of psychoneurosis endured as well as men with no previous history of psychological symptoms. Given a long enough commitment to battle of any severity, all men were potential psychiatric casualties: "Every man has his breaking point."

In World War II the individual at highest risk for psychiatric breakdown in battle was the line infantryman or the dismounted armored infantryman (Mericle, 1946). The situation that most predisposed to risk was intense static warfare conducted in an either offensive or defensive posture. The impact of psychiatric casualties on the ability to maintain force levels was great, particularly when we recognize that overall divisional and field army figures are somewhat misleading. The primary impact of psychiatric casualties was felt at the level of the line company, battalion, and regiment, those units actually engaged in direct combat. The overall European Army rate of 101 per thousand per annum is biased by the inclusion of data from the end of the Battle of the Bulge to the end of hostilities. This was a period when the generation of neuro-psychiatric (NP) casualties was extremely low because imminent victory was in sight. This bias masks the fact that individual line regiments often suffered annual rates as high as 1,600 per thousand per annum during the days or weeks of a heavy engagement.

These rates and patterns of psychiatric breakdown were incurred by troops that had been screened a number of times prior to commitment to battle. The Selective Service initially rejected 5,250,000 men, 1,686,000 of whom were excluded for emotional, mental, or educational disorders or deficiencies. Between 1942 and 1945, an additional 504,000 men were separated from the army on psychiatric or behavioral grounds (Ginzberg, 1959). In addition to these outright rejections and separations, a consistent process of weeding out individuals thought to be psychiatrically at risk took place throughout World War II (and during the Korean and Vietnamese conflicts as well).

At each stage, psychiatrists, other medical officers, and commanders arranged to have men transferred from combat units to service and support units, that is, from potential combat positions to noncombat positions. This weeding out process took place at training centers, in the initial divisional assignment, upon notification of embarkations, following debarkation and during time spent in the staging area, and immediately prior to deployment into battle.

Almost all World War II division psychiatrists cite such pre-combat screening as one of their regular roles. The population that broke down in combat did not represent a random cross-section of military personnel. It was a group that had been purged of its "weaker" personnel by the available psychiatric and administrative techniques of the times.

The overt neuropsychiatric casualty is only one category of losses that can be anticipated other than Wounded in Action (WIA) and Killed in Action (KIA) which will be generated by severe and sustained combat. Behavioral breakdown comes in many guises, ranging from death or wounding owing to behavioral lapses and errors of judgment (generated as a direct result of the psychophysiological deficits brought about by the combat reaction or combat fatigue) to increases in illnesses known to have a psychogenic or psychosomatic component, and, further, to increases in rates of injury and physical illness. Illnesses that are preventable through volitional behavior such as frostbite and malaria also increase. These types of illnesses are often generated by stress and are recognized as collateral or secondary psychiatric casualties. From a psychodynamic point of view, the soldier in combat is caught between two contending and overwhelming forces: the need to stay and do his duty, and the desire to escape the life-threatening terror of the battlefield. During World War II, going absent without leave (AWOL) was the most obvious way to escape battle, but somatic complaints or minor injuries were more legitimate ways of escaping battle for hours or even days. The subtlest of these losses were those in which the individual became a physical casualty for psychological reasons. This situation was indirectly examined by division psychiatrist R. L. Swank and W. E. Marchand (1946) who developed a model of the relationship of combat exhaustion to combat efficiency in Normandy in 1944.

The initial period of combat saw acute combat reactions mostly in the form of severe anxiety states. This ended after four to five days, and the soldier started to reach his period of maximum efficiency which peaked at twenty-one days and lasted approximately a week afterward. Then:

The first symptom of combat exhaustion made its appearance at about D plus 25 to D plus 30 days in most soldiers. This was an abnormal fatigability which could no longer be relieved by periods of rest up to forty-eight hours. The fear reactions, so noticeable early in combat and so successfully controlled during the period of high efficiency in battle, reappeared more frequently and were quelled with less success. Unconsciously, the soldier lost confidence in

himself. This was clearly shown in his reactions toward various battle stimuli. He began to lose the fine points of discrimination in which he prided himself. He could no longer tell the difference between friendly and enemy artillery and mortar fire and referred to all as the fabulous "eight-eight."
To all these stimuli his reactions became excessive often to the point where they were harmful. He became overcautious; he stayed close by or in his slit trench whenever possible; he walked rather than rode in a vehicle so that he would be able to get to cover more readily; and he became a follower rather than a leader.

After forty to forty-five days of combat in Normandy, the authors note:

. . . The soldier was slow witted; he was slow to comprehend simple orders, directions and techniques, and he failed to perform even life-saving measures such as digging in quickly. Memory defects became so extreme that he could not be counted upon to relay a verbal order.

The soldier killed or wounded as a result of such stress and situationally induced deficits was seldom counted as a psychiatric casualty. The actual number of these soldiers is unknown, but we may hazard the guess that they presented a significant proportion of our killed and wounded.

The general relationship between noncombat injuries and severity and intensity of combat was established over and over again in both World War II and Korea. Injuries with particularly significant behavioral components that are dependent in great part on volitional behavior, for example, frostbite, also closely followed the curve of combat intensity. Like relationships were seen with incidences of malaria in the Pacific and with cold injury in the Korean conflict.

Breakdown in battle takes many forms, some of which are interchangeable. Severe combat that produces few combat psychiatric casualties as labeled by the Medical Department produces compensatorily large numbers of personnel withdrawn from battle for frostbite, illness, or light injury, as well as AWOL and self-inflicted wounds. The symptoms have many different diagnostic names but are basically equivalent—critical combat personnel are not available for or capable of performing their duty for varying lengths of time. Most may be restored to duty, whether NP casualty, light injury, or illness, but in each case, for periods varying from twenty-four hours to several weeks, critical combat personnel are not available to engage the enemy.

History has not been made irrelevant by changes in the human species, by drugs, by the technologies of warfare, or by changes in the soldier's capacity to adapt to the battlefield. Low-intensity war fought against an opponent with limited weaponry such as the Vietnam conflict indeed produced fewer psychiatric casualties than previous conflicts. The cause, however, lay in the nature of the war and not in changes in either selection, quality of personnel, or technology since World War II. The proof of this lies in the Arab-Israeli War of 1973. In this war, which featured high-intensity sustained combat, 10 percent of all Israeli casualties were psychiatric. Few were cases of combat fatigue, that is, the erosion of men by moderately intense battle across time such as characterized World War II. Most were classified as combat reactions, that is, a more rapid breakdown of men by sustained combat of high intensity for briefer periods of time. The war, after all, lasted only three weeks. Breakdown patterns, however, followed the same rules with respect to severity of battle as measured by KIA/WIA figures.

Battle, then, has devastating effects on its participants. If it is sufficiently severe, intense, and long in duration, it will ultimately break everyone committed to it. That is a simple enough message and one with few redeeming virtues for the miltiary planner. However, World War II provided us with another set of phenomena and data of critical importance to leaders of ground combat forces.

Although all men were ultimately at risk for breakdown, units, divisions, regiments, and battalions were not equally exposed. Risk changed with time as divisions suffered their baptism of severe combat, as did the 88th Division at Volterra where NP casualties reached 32 percent of WIA. NP casualties accounted for only 22 percent of WIA in equivalently heavy combat on the Gothic line just three months later, with a large number of those casualties coming from new replacements. Divisions responded differently. Green divisions, meeting powerful enemy forces for the first time, tended to have high numbers of NP casualties as in Tunisia at the battles of the Kasserine and Faid passes. There, NP casualties reached levels as high as 35 percent of all casualties, combat and noncombat.

Other units tended to have significantly lower rates than their sister divisions or regiments. In thirty-six days of fighting at the Gustav Line, NP casualties reached 13 percent of WIA in the 34th Division. The 91st Division, engaged in lighter battle at the Cecina River, suffered only a third as many WIA, and yet NP casualties reached 33 percent of the number wounded in thirty-five days. The 91st was a green division, whereas the 34th was known as a division of particularly high morale whose psychiatric casualty rates were persistently below those of fellow units. An equally powerful differentiation is seen when we contrast the psychiatric casualty rates of elite units in World War II, the airborne divisions, with those of the other divisions at which we have looked. In no engagement for which data are available did the rate of neuropsychiatric casualties exceed 5.6 percent of WIA in any of the three airborne divisions deployed in European Theater of Operations (ETO). Other units demonstrated equivalent differences. The 442 Regimental Combat Team, comprised primarily of Nisei from Hawaii and relocation centers, and the most decorated unit in the U.S. Army, had almost no psychiatric casualties throughout the Italian Campaign.

Contrast is provided by the 24th and 43rd Divisions in the Pacific theatre, both of which had major and chronic problems with NP casualties. The 24th Division, which had been responsible for the defense of Oahu during Pearl Harbor, seemed to function as if it were under the perpetual stigma of failure and incompetence. In addition to large numbers of psychiatric casualties in its first campaign, the division was characterized by an unusual amount of homosexuality throughout its deployment.

The 43rd Division lost almost 10 percent of its *total* strength as NP casualties in New Georgia. The division had been characterized by poor morale and by leadership problems. In combat, psychiatric breakdown was contagious, and mass breakdown occurred among small groups such as infantry squads. The relationship between the pattern of breakdown and the division's organization problems is indicated by the fact that the number evacuated from each company, or similar unit, was found to be in direct proportion to the number of unit leaders evacuated.

It is obvious that the power of battle to generate behavioral breakdown and nonavailability of unwounded personnel for duty is not absolute. This is demonstratably true in high-intensity, high-lethality, contemporary main force conventional warfare. In the 1973 war the Israelis reported almost no psychiatric casualties in elite airborne and certain other forces, regardless of the intensity of combat.

Certain mediating factors enable men to ward off psychological breakdown and to demonstrate lower levels of temporarily disabling physical disease and injury and significantly lower levels of injuries and diseases with a behavioral component. For example, in the Vietnam conflict Australian forces had much lower rates of malaria than American troops in the same areas. The Australians rigorously adhered to their health and anti-malarial regimes in a way that the Americans did not.

Forces conducive to breakdown in battle are for the most part inherent in the structure of battle itself. The primary and most powerful force is the enemy whose mission and intent is to break his opponent by creating an environment in which organized, coordinated, and effective combat behavior ceases to be a possibility for the members and units of that opposing force. The enemy controls a number of stressors on the battlefield beginning with the array of weaponry and the tactical and strategic doctrines that govern their use. The enemy also has a great measure of control over the severity and duration of combat, and the size of the zone of lethality to which one's forces are subjected. Thus, the enemy influences the configuration of the front and rear of the combat zone, as well as the proportion of forces subjected to the direct stresses of the combat zone. This is true particularly of the peculiarly stressful impact of heavy indirect fire, a factor consistently associated with large numbers of psychiatric and nonbattle casualties. Support troops at Anzio, for example, where the entire beachhead was under regular enemy interdictory fire, had much higher than expected rates of psychiatric breakdown.

The Yom Kippur War of 1973 demonstrated that logistic troops in the Israeli Defense Force (IDF) were at peculiarly high risk for psychiatric casualties in proportion to physical casualties. Discussions with IDF medical and personnel indicated that the bulk of these casualties took place in units that were subject to enemy medium- and long-range artillery fire as well as air attack.

The high-intensity, sustained group warfare projected as a scenario for the immediate future in Europe, and elsewhere, assumes a maximization of the factors that historically have led to breakdown in battle. This is expressed in terms of the doctrine of sustained echeloned attack, comprising nine to twelve pulses of combat per day (compared to the three or four pulses of extremely severe combat in World War II or Korea), with extensive and continual use of massed weapons of

THE HUMAN DIMENSION OF COMBAT BREAKDOWN

indirect fire that characterize strategic and tactical doctrine in Soviet and Warsaw Pact nations.

With the Israeli battles in both the Sinai and Golan as an introductory model, we could expect an initial battle of great severity, stress, and duration. The troops receiving this thrust would be engaged in continuous combat, with little sleep and little relief from the pressures of closing with the enemy. Green troops, as yet untried in combat, would receive initially severe battle exposure at levels of intensity and lethality that might be three to four times those of World War II. Many units would take initially high casualty rates. Men would require sustained and complete alertness, hour after hour, day after day, to meet the assaults of a well-organized and technologically sophisticated enemy. Rumors and ignorance would spread and lead to misinterpretation of the actual tactical situation. Men would be surrounded by the dead and the mutilated. Tank crews would have to be reconstituted from survivors two or three times in the course of the opening engagements. Men would suffer chronic fatigue, watch friends be blown apart, be poorly fed, poorly hydrated, and desperately concerned about families and dependents.

This is neither an imaginative recitation of the horrors of war nor a set of fantasies about stress on the battlefield. These are the most commonly cited factors that operated on the individual to produce breakdown in World War II and Korea.

The basic set of factors that were perceived as countervailing to the vast array of battlefield forces operating to break men were of complex behaviors and attitudes usually categorized under the phrases "unit morale" or "group cohesion." Herbert Spiegel (1944) made the initial set of observations (for a psychiatrist) on the relationship of group cohesion or morale and the sustainability of men in battle during the Tunisian Campaign:

If abstract ideas—hate or desire to kill—did not serve as strong motivating forces, then what did serve them in that criticial time? What enabled them to attack, and attack, and attack week after week in mud, rain, dust and heat until the enemy was smashed? It seemed to me that the drive was more a positive than a negative one. It was love more than hate. Love manifested by 1) regard for their comrades who shared the same dangers, 2) respect for their platoon leader or company commander who led them wisely and backed them with everything at his command, 3) concern for their reputation with their commander and leaders, and 4) an urge to contribute to the task and success of their group and unit (p. 312).

In each case in which observers noted variation from the mean, at any level—battalion, regiment, division—given equivalent conditions of battle the differences could be accounted for by observable, and, in some cases, measurable, differences in group cohesion and unit morale. The overwhelming consensus of all observers was that the unit was the primary defender against or expediter of breakdown in battle. As Colonel A. J. Glass, the leading combat psychiatrist and theoretician of combat psychiatry in the U.S. Army in this century, put it in summing up the experience of World War I, World War II, and Korea:

Available epidemiological data indicated that the mental illness of troops in warfare, exclusive of psychotic disorders, is more significantly related to circumstances of the combat situation than to any personality attributes or characteristics of the individuals who are exposed to battle stress. Pertinent combat circumstances include the intensity and duration of battle which can be measured by the battle casualty rate and the days of continuous action. However, of equal importance in determining the frequency of psychiatric cases are less measurable elements of battle; to wit, the degree of support given the individual by buddies, group cohesiveness and leaders. These less tangible influences explain the marked differences that may occur in combat effectiveness and the frequency of psychiatric cases among units which are exposed to the same intensity and duration of battle (Glass, 1954).

Unfortunately, the hard-won knowledge that was developed out of military psychiatry and social and behavioral science was essentially lost except for the armed forces. Medicine, in general, and psychiatry and psychology reverted to their peacetime ideologies, practices, and therapies based on the individual as the unit of predisposition, risk, and cure. The disease model that underlies most of Western thought has been based on a view of the individual organism as a bounded and autonomous entity whose unique history and physiology interacting in exposure to environmental agents determines the response of both body and mind, as well as the impact of psychological stress on the body.

It was not until the mid- to late 1960s that a rising school of psychosocial epidemiologies led by such men as Cassel, Cobb, and Brown began to assay the effects of group membership on mediating stress and altering risk for disease. At the heart of their work is the concept of social support—that is, the presence or absence of a network of people and institutions which the individual sees as concerned about his or her well-being and survival. Its ultimate rationale is sociobiological. Men evolved as members of structured and ordered social groups, and indeed sociality and membership in a hierarchy are part of the fundamental definition of "being human."

Because nature tends to be parsimonious, numerous adaptational advantages apparently accrue to the individual from group membership and group support. Recent research in the relationship of stress, social support systems, and physical and mental disease indicates that such group affiliations play a major role in protecting the individual against breakdown, illness, and even death in the presence of psychosocial and environmental stress.

Contemporary studies document the strength of the relationship between the social support system—the other individuals and groups to which the individual is bonded—and disease, mental illness, and death. The exact mechanisms through which such mediation is effected remains unknown at present. The most common set of hypotheses involves the effects of stress on nervous, hormonal, and immunological control systems in the body. Laboratory work with animals and with tissue cultures has demonstrated that psychosocial as well as physical stress (1) modifies control systems; (2) severely alters hormonal balances; and (3) can suppress the level of activity of the immune system. In this model social supports are believed to operate to dampen and mitigate such effects on the body's control systems, thus shoring up its resistance to breakdown.

In World War II, the Korean War, and the Vietnam War, the U.S. Army was rich in both personnel and time. Nonbattle and psychiatric casualties could be compensated, and resources existed to provide large numbers of replacements for units suffering high casualty rates. In the Korean and Vietnam conflicts, both of which were perceived as limited in scope and required only modest allocations of the nation's substance in manpower, group cohesiveness was traded for rapid rotation. These wars threatened the physical integrity of neither the army nor the nation. The soldier's behavior was organized by a perception of "his war," that is, one that would occupy a fixed period of time and that he would quit if he survived that fixed period. In each of these wars, however, time existed to forge armies and to forge the bonds of the small groups that comprised those armies. There were palpable enemies, months of training and anticipation of combat, and long periods in transit during which men could bond to their units and their fellows.

The soldier's bonds to other men, bonds which he perceived as time limited, were more instrumental in the sense of being more overtly discussed, than those based on self-interest and seen as transient. Operationally, the behavior that men exhibited, at least during the first nine months of a tour in line units, differed not at all from the group bonding behavior exhibited by line troops in World War II. In the last three months of their tours, however, men tended to withdraw from close relationships with others in their units and to lose combat efficiency and willingness to engage in combat as they moved into a low-risk mode prior to DEROS.

Much of the cohesion that existed during these wars was built on the battlefield. For the most part, the tempo of battle was such that the final welding of squad, platoon, and company was effected during the initial week to ten days of commitment to combat. Often, however, too much emphasis is placed on the function of battle in creating group cohesion. In its initial deployment to battle, unless the unit is shattered by overwhelming enemy strength, the cohesion provided by battle is only the icing on the cake of the unit's preexisting cohesion and morale.

A critical issue for any army in assuring readiness for potential main force war is the establishment of predeployment strong cohesion and high morale to ensure the minimization of psychiatric and noncombat casualties. Among the more salient reasons are:

1. Lack of time for the creation of strong group morale and powerful formal and informal bonds in the period between enemy attack and massive commitment of troops. This period is measured in minutes, hours, and, at most, days in the event of a ground conflict with Warsaw Pact forces.
2. Limited manpower resources during the initial and critical phases of such a war will mandate maximum conservation of personnel. This must be accomplished in order to ensure adequate force levels and adequate cadres for the swift reconstitution of units. NP and nonbattle casualties must be kept to a minimum.
3. The team structures dictated by both present and future weaponry mandate

THE HUMAN DIMENSION OF COMBAT BREAKDOWN   19

the existence of well-bonded and organized work groups if they are to be used with optimum efficiency and effect.

4. The reception and destruction of attacking enemy forces, superior in both numbers and quantity of equipment, require high cohesion and morale on the part of the defending forces if they are to hold and destroy them.
5. In high-intensity conventional warfare, forces involved in sustained operations will be subjected to an intensity and density of battle and lethality, for longer periods of time, and on a greater scale than has ever been seen before. History has shown us that this structure of battle is capable of producing the greatest number of psychiatric and nonbattle casualties.
6. Although cohesion and morale do not correlate with technical performance, as *The American Soldier* (Stouffer et al., 1949) and other studies demonstrate, they do correlate with military performance in the sense of effectively maintaining the organized group at its tasks even in face of severe battle stress.

Given (1) the anticipated size and lethality of a projected assault; (2) the number of casualties by death and wounding that will disrupt the bonds of the average military unit; and (3) the fact that the most powerful precipitant of psychiatric breakdown in battle is the death of a man's closest buddy, is the question of maintaining high levels of group cohesiveness and unit morale operationally important? In this context, it is important to remember that the cohesion that protected men from breakdown, the morale that shielded them, at least in part from the stresses of the battlefield, was not simply built on affective bonds of comradely love between soldiers. It was built within the framework of the institutions of the military and of the human organization provided by those institutions.

The argument is a critical one. Interpersonal bonding is only one of the forces that keep men in battle. The weight of the bonding and its positive effect is highly dependent on the structure and organization of the unit. It is dependent on the ability of the unit as a structure and a set of ideas, a culture, to maintain men in their roles as soldiers. No matter how strong personal attachments are, if they are not consonant with the structure of the military unit, the role of the soldier, and the division of labor in the unit and mission performance, they will not be enough to maintain men in battle.

In this context it is important to reiterate a series of fundamental truths. Armies, divisions, brigades, and battalions do not possess cohesion, nor do they possess morale. In terms of the social structure of the military, only teams, squads, platoons, and companies achieve cohesion. The only people in a brigade who are members of a division are brigade staff and so on. The larger institutional membership of the men in the squads, platoons, and companies is, at best, nominal, and the men achieve this membership only through the roles their company officers and senior NCOs play as their representatives to higher levels.

The social universe of the enlisted soldier revolves around his squad and platoon and extends only to the boundary of his company. Battalion, brigade, and division activities may affect the soldier's morale and cohesiveness, but the fundamental behaviors, roles, and attitudes that determine whether or not each small group is cohesive are decided at squad, platoon, and company level. The institutional boundaries and constraints that will have determining power on group cohesion and morale are essentially those that are defined at company level and below.

It is at the squad and platoon level that group integrations are achieved, group norms are defined, and standards of behavior are informally set. At this level the relationship of informal standards of behavior to institutionally defined standards and need is determined, and, consequently, much of the unit's military effectiveness is defined.

There has been much conflict in recent years over the continued importance of the primary group to soldiers in battle. The question that has been raised is, does the primary group as locus of support—that is, the squad or platoon as a grouping of eight to twenty affectively bonded men supporting and controlling behavior—actually exist? Was it a time- and culture-bond artifact of soldiers during World War II, or an analytic misinterpretation based on the prevalent scientific ideologies of the time? Such an accusation was recently made in respect to Shils and Janowitz' analysis of the role of primary group affective bonds in maintaining group cohesion and commitment to combat in the Wermacht (Shils and Janowitz, 1948). Much of the recent conflict has been precipitated by observations in Vietnam which present an essentially economic model of combat relationships based on self-interest.

Were the differences in perceived pattern of group affiliation attributable to the policy of rotation, observer interpretation, or a combination of these factors? Certainly, as has been indicated, the rotation policies in both Korea and Vietnam had major effects on group bonding and cohesion. During these wars one entered the group with full knowledge that it was explicitly time-bound for oneself. This knowledge of necessity defines relationships as having a more economic or instrumental, that is, self-serving, aspect that is founded on the sure perception that the group will of necessity be dissolved at a given point in time.

Time-bound instrumental relationshps that are based on self-interest have no less supportive power than those entered into out of "pure" affect. Careful study of data from World War II and Korea and Vietnam demonstrates little difference in the actualities and operations of the bonding process. In all three wars for the combat soldier the combat group was a group of "potential buddies," and the primary group existed for him in terms of his buddy, or buddies, of the moment.

The group's power, then, lay in its capacity to provide an array of individuals who were potential buddies. The continual economic or self-nature of a large aspect of this relationship has been described by wounded veterans:

You know the men in your outfit. You have to be loyal to them. The men get close-knit together. They like each other—quit their petty bickering and having enemies. They depend on each other—wouldn't do anything to let the rest of them down. They'd rather be killed than do that. They begin to think the world of each other. It's the main thing that keeps a guy from going haywire. The worst thing a solider can have is to see other guys dropping. Sticking together is the important thing—with someone in command to push them along—everybody's afraid.

or

The fellows don't want to leave when they're sick. They're afraid to leave their own men—the men they know. They don't want to get put in a different outfit. Your own outfit—they're the men you have confidence in. It gives you more guts to be with them (Stouffer et al., 1949, p. 236).

The instrumental or self-interest motive plays as significant a role as affection in the buddy relationship, a characteristic that in no way lessens or demeans the buddy relationship. The relationship essentially consists of an economic exchange of social support, with each party dedicated to preserving the survival of the other as the necessary aspect of the exchange as much as, if not more than, affection or comradely love.

The shorter the time period allocated to a set of relationships within a group and a unit the more instrumental and self-serving it will appear to the observer. In terms of group structure, the peacetime analogue to combat has always been Basic Training, a time of extremely high stress, involving radical environmental changes and an evoking strong group cohesion.

Despite the fact that the ex-trainee will seldom even remember the names of his buddies some weeks or months after the end of Basic Training, during the stressful parts of the process he credits them with his ability to endure and successfully negotiate training. Thus, in terms of providing support and the sustaining aspect of affective bonds, for the critical period of its existence the transient grouping of basic trainee functions no differently than "primary groups" did in World War II.

To be militarily effective then the squad or platoon must exhibit a primary pattern of bonding in terms of skills and reliability as soldiers. The potentiality for these bonds being created is diffused throughout the squad or platoon, and, as some sociometric studies have shown, there are many one-way as well as mutual choices of buddies. The squad is an open but interlocking network, with the majority of choices for linkage based on technical skill and enough room for other choices based on other personal attributes. For such cohesion to be truly protective, the unit must also have good morale.

High morale comprehends a number of factors, all of which ultimately define the term "military cohesion":

1. Trust and confidence in one's fellow soldiers.
2. Trust and confidence in the competence of and fairness of one's NCOs.
3. Trust and confidence in the competence and fairness of one's officers.
4. Trust and confidence in one's equipment.
5. Trust and confidence in the technical abilities and military power of the unit.
6. A sense of support from significant others in the civil community.
7. The belief in one's ability to defeat the enemy.
8. Trust and confidence in one's own combat ability.

Many other factors could be adduced, but in essence they all add up to bonding with one's fellows, trust in one's leaders and followers, support from home, and confidence in the unit's power.

CONCLUSION

The problem of creating and maintaining cohesive, high-morale groups in the combat arms and combat support services is critical to the maintenance and reconstitutability of ground forces in a high-intensity war. The fundamental problems are conceptual and perceptual, and interact with the ongoing structure of the military to create units that are more or less cohesive and that have greater or less morale. If this is so, then the difficulties involved in establishing and maintaining cohesive, high-morale groups must be resolved in the realms of ideas and behaviors rather than in questions of selection for marginal differences in personnel qualities. The resolutions developed must be conceptual and philosophical, and must involve the military's view of itself as an institution, encompassing its organization and above all its end goals and missions.

The structures and relationships required to achieve these ends and to ensure endurance and reconstitutability in battle must become a major question for commanders, staffs, and policymakers. Which concepts and behaviors should be expected and required from those officers and senior and midlevel NCOs who ensure the continuity of ideas and patterns of relationship within the formal structure of the military? To what ends should they be encouraged, trained, and graded to help ensure the recognition of the critical relationships between the behavior of representatives of the formal structure at company and lower levels, and the cohesion of the military as a whole? What special attention must be paid to the critical transition points in the life of the service member as he moves from the high motivation of the training environment to his first duty station? These points of specialization, from training to permanent duty or from unit to unit, represent critical events in which the unit may determine the strengths of its future corporate bonds, both formal and informal, as well as the power of the correlation between the two. If our culture has provided personnel unskilled in the art of being members of corporate groups and unskilled in recognizing the relationship of one's own self-interest to that of the group, perhaps we must give more thought to training teams and groups than to individual skills alone. If good units require the capacity for rapid development of diffuse buddy relationships, perhaps we must train men to be replacements as well as to be members of teams and squads. Once battle begins, an army limited to its personnel resources has little trial-and-error time to shake itself down into cohesive units.

Despite the existence of technical aids, the problems involved are not those that are simply amenable to technical fixes. These "technical fixes" will avail us nothing unless they are designed to achieve better cohesion and morale, that is, trust, confidence, mutual respect, belief in self and unit, and mutual support at team, squad, platoon, and company levels. Hence, these "cultural" aspects of an army must first be addressed if men are to learn to sustain their sanity amid the horrors of the battlefield. Even then, many will be unable to do so, and the problem of psychiatric breakdown under fire will remain with us at least for the foreseeable future and perhaps forever.

REFERENCES

Appel, J. W., and Beebe, G. W. (1946). Preventive psychiatry: an epidemiological approach. *Journal of the American Medical Association*, *131*, August 18, 1469-1475.

Ginzberg, Eli. (1959). *The lost divisions*. New York: Columbia University Press.

Glass, A. J. (1954). *Observations upon the epidemiology of mental illness in troops during warfare*. Symposium on Preventive and Social Psychiatry, WAIR-NRC, Washington, D.C.: U.S. Government Printing Office.

Mericle, E. W. (1946). The psychiatric and tactical situations in an armored division. *Bulletin of the U.S. Army Medical Department*, *6*, 325-334.

Musser, J.A., and Stengers, R. (1972). A medical and social perception of the Vietnam veteran. *Bulletin of the New York Academy of Medicine*.

Shils, Edward and Janowitz, Morris. (1948). Cohesion and disintegration in the German Wehrmact in W.W. II. *Public Opinion Quarterly*, 12.

Spiegel, H. X. (1944). Preventive psychiatry with combat troops. *American Journal of Psychiatry*, *101* (November).

Stouffer, S. A. et al. (1949). *The American soldier*. 5 vols. Princeton, N.J.: Princeton University Press.

Swank, R. L., and Marchand, W. E. (1946). Combat neuroses: development of combat exhaustion. *Archives of Neurology and Psychology*, *55*, 236-247.

2
American Military Psychiatry

LAWRENCE INGRAHAM
and FREDERICK MANNING

Psychiatric battle casualties became commonplace in the wars of the twentieth century. Prior to the Russo-Japanese War of 1904–1905, such casualties were noted by military physicians, but never in sufficient numbers to constitute a military-medical problem.

American attempts to understand and respond to battle stress casualties have ranged from the positively brilliant to the positively pathetic. Twice in this century the American Army considered the problem solved, and twice, at the beginning of World War II and following Vietnam, it found the conventional wisdom wanting and either had to rediscover what had earlier been learned or had to abandon concepts that seemed at the time both elegant and self-evident. Understanding the American experience with these casualties requires considerations of the ever changing ecology of the modern battlefield as it responds to changes in technology, ideology, and scientific understanding.

The first question, then, is what is so special about twentieth-century warfare? From ancient times battlefields have epitomized terror, fear, chaos, slaughter, and cruelty. Winston Churchill (1933) provides an unforgettable picture of Marlborough's battlefields:

The views of the authors do not purport to reflect the positions of the department of the army or the department of defense. (Para 4-3, AR-360-5).

Sometimes two hundred thousand men fought for an afternoon in a space no longer than the London parks put together, and left the ground literally carpeted with maimed or slaughtered men. . . . In prolonged severe fighting the survivors of a regiment often stood for hours knee-deep amid the bodies of comrades writhing or forever still. In their ears rang the hideous chorus of the screams and groans of a pain which no anesthetic would ever soothe.

No one ever argued that battlefields were conducive to positive mental health. Yet few accounts exist of what we would now call a psychiatric battle casualty. In former times, one of the adversaries quickly perceived that the advantage lay with the other side and quite rationally refused to continue the battle. Commanders who lost control were often branded incompetents or cowards, but not mental cases; soldiers who froze in terror were forgiven because military unit discipline had collapsed. The battle stress casualties of the twentieth century were quite different. They appeared both before and after active conflict, and were members of units that continued to engage the enemy with military discipline intact. Why the paucity of combat stress reactions until recent times?

The reasons lie in the ecology of premodern battle and the conditions of life that raised those armies. Until the late nineteenth century, armies in the field spent most of their time on the move, sometimes in search of the enemy, but mostly to find food for soldiers and animals. A major campaign of a year or more might see only one or two real battles and a handful of skirmishes. A real battle might last only a few hours or a few days, at most, before the armies were forced to disengage to search again for food and water resupply. There was terror, to be sure, but brief terror, rigidly controlled by the logistics required to sustain engagement. Armies seldom fought in the winter and never at night. Once the armies disengaged, soldiers could look forward to days, weeks, or months without the horrors of battle.

The structure of battle also shielded frail individuals from psychological assault. The ancients recognized that the rational response to battlefield terror was to run away. To preclude this all too human and rational response, they organized the line of battle with comrades shoulder to shoulder so that the collective was far stronger than isolated individuals. Units were recruited from the same villages, and friends were placed near friends to increase the probability that individual soldiers would not run away and disgrace themselves before their peers. As long as the line held, the individual soldier could be counted on to do his duty; it would have taken a brave man indeed to run away. When the line or the square broke, all was lost, for no commander could hope for many individuals strong enough to stand and fight despite their fear. Those few who could became the stalwart heroes of legend and song, heroes precisely because their actions were so atypical.

Brief battles fought in closed formations with weapons sufficiently inaccurate to generate many casualties therefore protected premodern armies from what we now know as battle stress reactions. The chief psychological problem of earlier armies was one of group psychology: mass panic, not individual breakdown. To be sure, these armies must have known psychiatric disease; after all, psychosis is not new to this century, but such cases did not present much of a military problem. Psychotics were simply driven from the encampments and left to wander among the ravaged populace. After the army had eaten everything in sight and moved on, there were lots of folks wandering around in a daze. The few psychotic soldiers joined army stragglers and civilians in eking out, as best they could, a life that was nasty, brutish, and short.

In the mid- to late-nineteenth century, improved transporation, manufacturing, and weapons technology, especially the rifled bore, changed the ecology of the battlefield, an ecology that had remained virtually unchanged for centuries. Armies no longer had to move in search of food. They remained in place with food and ammunition carted to them by steamboats and railroads. This apparent boon to armies was no blessing for their soldiers, however.

The American Civil War provides the first instance of individual psychological disturbances as a military problem. Civil War surgeons reported cases of depressed spirits, listlessness, and a longing for home which they termed nostalgia. Such cases were most prevalent among soldiers who had not yet experienced battle, who had not yet taken to the field in long road marches, but who were restricted to training camps and engaged in close order drill and the tedium of garrison life. Not many cases were reported, the chief military medical problems being surgical with attendant infections, but it is significant to note that once a conscript army stood still without the need for constant foraging, soldiers evidenced psychological distress.

The treatment of mentally ill soldiers also changed during the Civil

War. Northern citizens took exception to the past practice of simply cashiering mentally ill soldiers from the army to fend for themselves. Penniless, naked, and deranged ex-soldiers were viewed as a threat to public health and a safety, rather than just another nuisance attendant to the scourge of war. Citizens insisted that their government take responsibility for mentally ill soldiers, and St. Elizabeth's Hospital in Washington, D.C., was used to meet this need (Deutsch, 1944).

In the latter half of the nineteenth century, considerable progress was made in getting the mentally ill off the streets. Both the states and the federal government maintained asylums for the mentally ill. Physicians in these institutions also made progress in classifying the variety of derangements, creating rudimentary explanatory theories, and evolving treatment regimes. By the early twentieth century, psychiatry had emerged as one of the most promising and intellectually exciting of the new medical specialties.

Taxonomy was the keystone of nineteenth-century life science. What Linaeus had done for biology and Mendelyeev had accomplished in chemistry, Emile Kraeplin was applying to mental illnesses. New theories of natural selection and of genetic heritability provided the promise of dynamic explanation applied to static classification. It is not hard to imagine, then, the excitement in America over reports from the European War of yet another disease to add to the growing taxonomy of mental illness.

WORLD WAR I

Bailey, Williams, and Komora (1929) report that American neurologists and psychiatrists eagerly read the reports from the European battlefields:

From the earliest days of the fighting at Mons, stories had come to the United States of strange new diseases apparently having their origin in the stress and special horror of modern warfare and presenting problems in treatment and prevention that baffled the medical organizations of the armies that later were to become our allies (p. 1).

Even making allowances for exaggeration and imprecision in lay reports, it seemed obvious that this new type of casualty resulted from the inability of human beings to withstand the effects of high explosives, most notably artillery, even though their units had not panicked and they had escaped bodily injury. Descriptions of these "shell-shock" cases varied widely and included "staring eyes, violent tremors, a look of terror, and blue, cold extremities. Some were deaf, and some were dumb, others were blind or paralyzed" (Bailey, Williams, and Komora, 1929, p. 2).

By 1917 a coalition of mental health professions had been organized under the rubric of the National Committee for Mental Hygiene. The committee volunteered expert consultation to the army surgeon general and assisted by studying the neuropsychiatric needs of the American Army. It also developed plans for psychiatric hospital units to manage the expected surge of war neuroses.

The etiology of shell shock was indeed puzzling. The name "shell shock" derived from early assumptions that the brain had indeed been shocked by repeated exposure to high explosives, and the symptoms were evidence of neurological impairment. Two lines of evidence forced abandonment of this hypothesis. First, patients with head wounds and central nervous system damage seldom exhibited the symptoms; the disorder was almost invariably a malady of the unwounded. Second, prisoners of war evidenced no symptoms despite enduring the same shelling as their captors. The explanation, therefore, had to be mainly psychological, not neuropathological.

Evidence for the psychological hypothesis was more consistent. First, the symptoms in many cases resembled those seen in civilian practice, but colored, to be sure, in distinctive ways by the precipitating events of war. Second, studies of medical histories of returned Canadian soldiers revealed evidence of mental disease or strong neuropathic trends prior to their enlistments. Third, a study of American troops on the Mexican border revealed an incidence of mental disease in the army three times higher than, for example, New York State during the same period of time. The obvious conclusions of the Americans in 1917 was that shell shock was a direct consequence of the constitutional makeup of individuals exposed to shell fire, and that the best way to prevent functional war neuroses was psychiatric screening of army recruits.

Both conclusions were wrong, as the World War II experience was to show in tragic detail. In 1917, however, they seemed self-evident. Why? How did responsible, dedicated scientists and practitioners miss the central lesson: combat stress reactions are normal reactions to abnormal circumstances? The answer lies in the background and training of the consultants to the army surgeon general, the treatment plan instituted in the American Expeditionary Force (AEF) (which was correct in every detail), the experiences of the allied armies, and the brevity of American participation in active combat.

The consultants to the surgeon general were the specialists in abnormal psychology and mental disease who were superintendents of large state mental hospitals. When they reviewed the Canadian medical histories, they found predisposing factors and evidence (often to only slight degrees) of mental disorders that must have been entirely consistent with the thousands of records they had reviewed in their own hospitals. Without adequate control groups or knowledge of the distribution of such factors in a nonhospitalized (normal) population, they had no way of checking their logic.

Furthermore, the army in 1916 was far behind the civilian sector in the application of the new psychiatric knowledge. The dramatic prevalence of mental disease in Pershing's army in Mexico and the limited treatment facilities available to the army generally impressed the consultants. They were correct in recommending improved treatment opportunities in an institution where little or no treatment was available. They were correct in recommending more careful screening of recruits at induction stations where modern psychiatric criteria were not being applied at all.

Finally, their recommendations for preventing and treating war neuroses were entirely consistent with the experiences of the Allied armies. Dr. Thomas Salmon, a member of the National Committee on Mental Hygiene, visited England in 1917 to learn at first hand of the British and French experiences with war neuroses. Neither of these armies had initially excluded recruits with demonstrable psychopathic tendencies or even histories of hospitalization for insanity, and neither army was prepared for the great numbers of mental patients that subsequently entered the medical systems. Foremost among Salmon's recommendations to the Americans were the "rigid exclusion of all insane, feeble-minded, psychopathic, and neuropathic individuals" from the American Army, and the provision for entire military hospitals devoted to treating neuropsychiatric cases.

Salmon also recommended adoption of the Allied practice of forward treatment of battle stress casualties. Early in the war the British had evacuated their shell-shock casualties across the channel to the homeland. Very few ever returned to duty. As the political climate in

France deteriorated, the French were forced to treat their casualties near the firing line where significant numbers recovered and were returned to their units (Hausman and Rioch, 1967). The British then adopted the principle of forward treatment, which consisted of rest, light duty in a military rather than a hospital environment, and encouragement with the expectation that the soldiers would soon rejoin their comrades.

The American Army adopted Salmon's recommendations. Recruit screening procedures were enacted, and psychiatrists were assigned to combat divisions where they continued vigorous efforts to weed out the unfit. In combat, division psychiatrists endeavored to employ the principles of forward treatment. On the whole they were successful, but the character of the war had changed by the time American troops were committed to combat. The Allied armies were out of the trenches and on the move.

By May 1918 American physicians had learned that the natural response of a combat army was to free itself of its sick and wounded in the quickest way possible; evacuation to the rear. Treatment within the sound of the guns at fixed psychiatric hospitals became more and more impractical; the army moved forward while the psychiatrists too often remained far behind to treat their patients. Salmon and Fenton (1929) report: "Many difficulties arose unless the division psychiatrists scrutinized closely the flow of exhausted, concussed, and emotionally disturbed soldiers from the front and controlled to a certain extent their evacuation" (p. 305).

Having psychiatric expertise at the triage point was often impractical, however. Salmon and Fenton continued:

In consequence many hundreds of men suffering from exhaustion, concussion neurosis, fear, and other emotional states found themselves within a few days after leaving their organizations, in hospitals a hundred miles or more away from the front. Very few of these men ever returned to active duty.

The value of these experiences lay chiefly in the demonstration of the fact that American divisions (even after a careful selection), with the elimination of many psychopathic, mentally defective, and unstable men were capable of furnishing a large number of war neurotics under battle conditions, and that these patients were as resistant to treatment at points distant from the line as those in the armies of the French and British, upon whose experience our plan had been based (p. 306). The lesson was clear, but not sufficiently practiced to become an habitual part of subsequent army thinking and planning. The

A.E.F. suffered only 400 neuropsychiatric casualties and up to 75 percent were treated properly and returned to their units (p. 317).

Other important lessons were also introduced, though they would not be remembered twenty years later. Epidemiological risk factors for "war neurosis" stress casualties were identified:

1. Open warfare produced frequent casualties, but fewer than fighting that required soldiers to remain passive in the face of enemy bombardment.
2. The incoming whistling sounds, detonations, and consequent multilation caused by artillery fire generated psychiatric casualties; rifle and machine gun fire did not.
3. Many cases followed days of constant fighting with insufficient sleep, food, and water.
4. The last straw was most often an exploding shell that knocked the casualty to the ground, or the killing or wounding of a close comrade.
5. Cases came in many guises (e.g., among those evacuated as gas attack victims, many were suffering from only fatigue and emotional disturbance).

Treatment of victims was also no mystery; the difficulty was application behind an advancing army. Salmon and Fenton (1929, p. 313) list the following "Rules for Psychoneurosis Wards":

1. Each patient on admission to have a hot drink.
2. Each patient to have three full meals a day unless otherwise ordered.
3. Do not discuss the symptoms with the patient.
4. Be firm and optimistic in all your dealings with these patients.
5. No one is permitted in these wards unless assigned for duty.
6. The rapid cure of these patients depends on food, sleep, exercise, and the hopeful attitude of those who come in contact with them.

Salmon and Fenton went on to elaborate on the tenacity with which victims hung on to the shell-shock label, even when written on the initial evacuation card by an untrained corpsman. They went into considerable detail on measures necessary to maintain positive expectations that such cases would soon return to duty. First, these measures included emphasizing the glory and traditions of the division, regiment, and company, and encouraging each soldier to do his part. Second, evacuation to the rear was to be painted as total separation from "paternal officer and brother soldier, and a prelude to becoming that most unhappy of mortals, a lone casual" (p. 314). Third, accepting the physician's judgment that patients were indeed fit to return to their units was best accomplished in a group setting that again emphasized ties with comrades and the need to do one's part. The importance of the military group in sustaining individual functioning had been discovered but not yet recognized.

Salmon and Fenton above all emphasized simple procedures, often in the shelter of a barn or farmyard, and found no necessity for electroshock or hypnotic procedures. Sleep-inducing drugs had yet to be invented.

Unfortunately for the future, these treatment strategies were successfully employed in only one American division in the AEF. There were far fewer cases than expected owing to the breakout from the trenches, and the war ended too soon to drive home the central lessons of triage and treatment. The principal lesson taken from World War I was the necessity for even more vigorous personnel selection procedures to weed out the unfit. This view was reinforced during the interwar years by the high costs of veterans compensation for mental disability.

Within the army the war had produced important, postiive results. Army hospitals now had psychiatric wards and other facilities for treating the mentally ill in the most up-to-date manner, and had trained psychiatrists in uniform. By the time all this had transpired, however, the war had ended and there were no more shell-shock victims available for treatment. These physicians therefore turned their attention to abnormal reactions to normal environments, using the same theory and techniques as their civilian counterparts. They, too, saw the central triumph of World War I in terms of personnel selection, and joined the chorus calling for even higher enlistment standards which would eventually eliminate the mentally weak and defective from the army and save millions of dollars in veterans compensation.

WORLD WAR II

It has been suggested that American armed forces suffered grievously from stress casualties in the early stages of World War II because they forgot the lessons of World War I. We would argue that these enormous losses instead occurred because American psychiatry remembered the success of World War I all too well—but credited the wrong variables. Buoyed by a confidence derived from advances in the diagnosis and care of civilian mentally ill, the army's Medical Department too readily accepted full responsibility for prevention and treatment of ineffective but unwounded soldiers. The central theme of military psychiatry in World War II is, however, the steady retreat from the "stress + predisposition = mental illness" model which has so recently brought psychologically incapacitated soldiers under the wing of the Medical Department. The following sections cover some of the observations on psychiatric screening, characteristics of the victims, the nature of the affliction, and treatment efficacy which brought about this remarkable change in our conception of neuropsychiatric casualties.

Psychiatric Screening

Glass (1966), in summarizing the lessons which the profession of psychiatry learned from its World War II experiences, suggests that the most obvious lesson was the inability of psychiatric screening to effectively identify and thus eliminate the military's psychiatric problems at induction. Why the armed forces should have relied on psychiatric screening as heavily as they did is unclear. Glass (1966) sees it as "a logical extention of their denial or failure to appreciate the magnitude of the psychiatric problem in war" (p. 743), but Ginzberg et al. (1959) point to the recollection of World War I breakdowns as an important determinant of the armed services' interest in screening. Whatever the reasons, what is clear is that during the course of World War II, over 800,000 men were classified 4-F (unfit for military service) for mental or emotional reasons. As Table 2.1 shows, this is the result of a rejection rate more than fifteen times higher than the World War I rate. The same table, however, shows that, despite this evidence of considerably higher standards for selection in World War II, neuropsychiatric patients were admitted to military hospitals at twice the World War I rate, and separations for mental and emotional reasons also showed a nearly threefold increase over the World War I rate. Psychiatric problems, in fact, were the largest single category of disability discharges in World War II (Bartemeier et al., 1946). Although

Table 2.1
Men Rejected for Military Service and Enlisted Men Separated from the Army for Emotional or Mental Reasons, World War I and World War II

	Number		Rate per 100	
	WW I	WW II	WW I	WW II
Rejections[a]	68,000	877,000	4	55
Separations[a]	25,000	486,000	7	21
Admissions[b]	106,000	929,000	28	44

[a] from Karpinos & Glass (1966)
[b] from Appel (1966

it might be argued that lower selection standards might have resulted in still higher separation rates, that the psychiatric screening actually done was far from the state of the art, that retention standards were much higher in World War II, or that the physical and psychological demands on soldiers were much more severe in World War II, it is undeniable in the face of these data that psychiatric screening fell far short of solving the psychiatric casualty problem of modern war. Having said this, it must be admitted that little else unequivocal can be gleaned from the figures of Table 2.1. Admissions and discharges, for example, are subject to policy and administrative decisions quite independent of symptomatology and treatment efficacy (Brill, 1966; Appel, 1966). This is illustrated by Figures 2.1 and 2.2, which show monthly discharge and admission rates for neuropsychiatric conditions by the U.S. Army, 1942–1945. The sharp rises and falls in both sets of curves reflect changes in policy and criteria for admitting patients and discharging soldiers. War Department Circular No. 161, issued in July 1943, for example, eliminated the category of "limited service" and ordered the discharge of all men who did not meet induction standards. The resulting tidal wave of discharges led to Circular No. 293 in November, prohibiting medical officers from discharging psychiatric patients from the army if they were capable of rendering any useful service. Circular No. 370, reversing No. 293, was issued in September 1944, and No. 370 was itself rescinded in January 1945 as the Battle of the Bulge began, all of which are reflected in Figure 2.1.

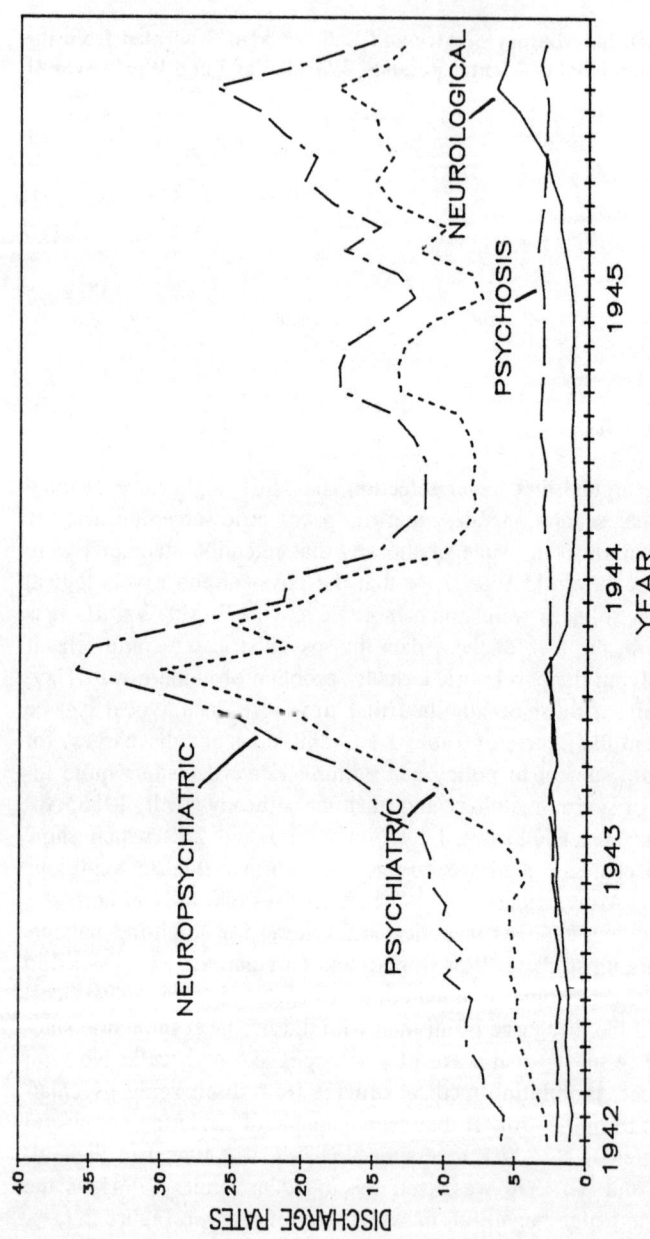

Figure 2.1
Discharge Rates of Enlisted Men for Neuropsychiatric Conditions, U.S. Army, by Year and Month, 1942–1945

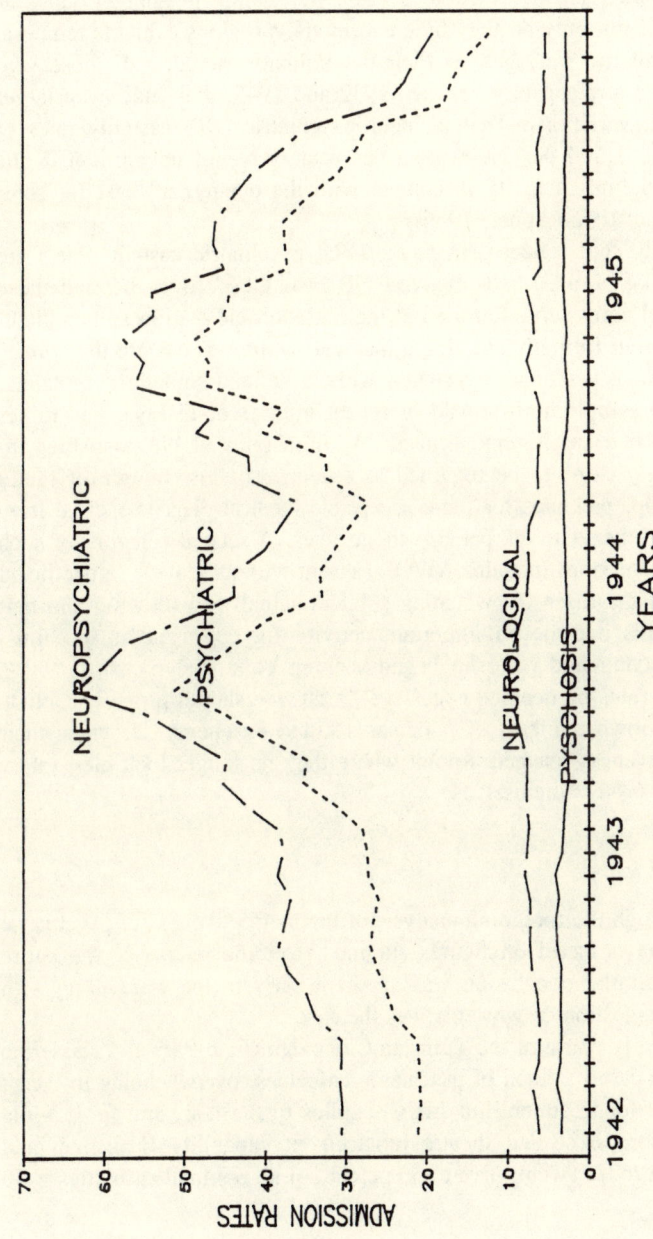

Figure 2.2
Admission Rates for Neuropsychiatric Disorders, U.S. Army, by Year and Month, 1942–1945

The rates shown in Table 2.1 are misleading in another sense as well, for not only do they hide enormous variations over the temporal course of the war, but, as their denominator includes all those who served in any capacity between 1942 and 1945, they hide even larger interunit variations. That is, neuropsychiatric (NP) casualty rates of 1,200 to 1,500 per 1,000 men per year were not uncommon in the rifle battalions actually in contact with the enemy, at least for short periods of time (Appel, 1966).

Finally, not reflected in any official psychiatric casualty rates are what Glass (1973) calls "covert NP casualties," even beyond those potential cases turned around at the battalion aid station and/or kitchens without formally entering a medical facility. These are the numerous combat personnel evacuated with ill-defined somatic complaints, residual symptoms from old or recent injuries or disease, and minor injuries like sprains and bruises. As high rates of NP casualties increasingly came to be regarded as evidence of low morale or faulty leadership, pressures for more acceptable medical diagnoses came from sources other than the patients themselves. A second category of such covert categories includes AWOL (absent without leave), self-inflicted wounds and diseases (watching soldiers actually swallowing anti-malarial pills became an important activity for commanders in Slim's Burma command once he began sacking commanders whose unit's malaria rates he deemed excessive). Last, we should properly include the unknown numbers of poor souls killed by enemy fire when their ineffectiveness reached a point where they no longer took elementary steps to protect themselves.

The Victims

Although the foregoing analysis of the ineffectiveness of psychiatric screening is based on figures summed over the course of the entire war, a similar conclusion was apparent early in the war, along with some suggestion of why this was the case.

The early phase of the Tunisian Campaign (Faid Pass and Kasserine Pass) produced a flood of psychiatric casualties, overwhelming the scant facilities for treatment hundreds of miles to the rear, and for a while evacuations exceeded theatre replacement capability (Hausman and Rioch, 1967). Twenty-five to 35 percent of all nonfatal casualties were psychiatric during this period, and only 3 percent were ever returned to combat duty (Drayer and Glass, 1973). By the beginning of the final battle for Tunisia, only two months later, however, psychiatrists had began to see that it was not merely predisposed "weaklings" who were breaking down, but to an increasing extent veteran combat troops who had already proven themselves in the difficult early going. Subsequent developments in the Mediterranean theatre confirmed this notion. In the two veteran divisions used in Sicily, 66 percent and 88 percent of the NP cases were veterans of the Tunisian Campaign who had not previously been hospitalized (Blesse, in Drayer and Glass, 1973). By the spring of 1944, following the Volturno, Rapido, and Cassino actions, it was more often old vets rather than new men who were coming in as psychiatric patients. Many were NCOs with strong combat records and decorations to prove it. It was on the Anzio beachhead that Sobel (cited in Glass and Drayer, 1973) coined the term "old sergeant syndrome," distinguished by "preexisting social and emotional adjustment of a high degree; marked sense of responsibility; and long combat in a responsible position" (p. 999). Although the victim did not claim to be sick, he noted more in sadness than anything else that he was changed, using phrases like "I'm no good anymore," "all burned out," or "I'll just get us all killed." In the face of such experiences, it was perhaps inevitable that both line and medical departments that should widely accept the notion that "every man has his breaking point." Appel (1966) cites a 1944 report which points out that in the North African theatre nearly all men in rifle battalions not otherwise disabled ultimately became psychiatric casualties. The author went on to estimate the limit of endurance for the average soldier as 200 to 240 aggregate combat days, although he concedes that most experienced line officers believed that most riflemen were noneffective, and perhaps even demoralizing to newer arrivals, after 140 to 180 days. In fact, Beebe and Appel (1958) estimated the "breaking point" of the average soldier at eighty to ninety combat days, based on the records of 2,500 frontline infantrymen sampled from all the principal infantry divisions of the Mediterranean and European theatres. They found that for each ten days of combat, from 3 to 10 percent of the men who still remained on duty broke down and were admitted to the hospital.

A concrete and far-reaching result of this realization that psychiatry was not just for the weak was a theatre directive issued in June of 1943 specifying that the only neuropsychiatric diagnosis to be employed for psychiatric casualties in the combat zone was "exhaustion." Drayer and Glass (1973), both of whom served as psychiatrists in North Africa, reported that "exhaustion" somehow made sense to all concerned, soldiers, line officers, and medical officers. (At this stage of the war the few psychiatrists in the theatre served as consultants or were concentrated in general and station hospitals far behind the lines.) Unlike "psychoneurosis" or "war neurosis," exhaustion carried no connotation of weakness and no implication of chronicity. We will return to the implications of this change for psychiatry as well as for the army, in the section on the nature of psychiatric casualties. For the moment we merely add that a parallel, though probably not independent, development was taking place in the Air Force, where the notion that only "weaklings" became NP casualties was a nonstarter, owing to the thoroughness of the pilot selection process. In fact, emotional problems were far from unknown among prewar peacetime fliers, and flight surgeons had spawned such terms as "flying fatigue" and "aero-asthenia" (Armstrong, 1939). The war only increased the opportunity to study these emotional reactions, and although psychiatrists quickly saw that they were by no means unique to fliers, they were forced to deal with the fact that the term "neurosis" carried more than a little stigma, which both flier and flight surgeon were loath to apply to the highly selected flying personnel. The result was the adoption of the term "operational fatigue" for "those cases of psychoneurosis which resulted from the stress of hazardous or combat flying" (Brill, 1966). This distinction had real significance for fliers (e.g., flight pay continued for personnel grounded with "operational fatigue," but not for those grounded because of "neurosis" of any sort), but its long-term significance lay in the fact that, like "exhaustion" and "combat fatigue," and the notion that every man had his breaking point, it symbolized the inadequacy of the "stress + predisposition = mental illness" model. If relatively normal soldiers or even pilots were susceptible, and the result was something that demanded a nonpsychiatric label, surely "predisposition" and "mental illness" were being used in far broader ways than originally intended. Still further observations on the nature of the NP casualty's disability only made this inadequacy even clearer.

Nature of the Affliction

History shows that there is no simple set of symptoms common to all wars, all psychiatric casualties, or even all phases of a given casualty's dysfunction. Many of these changes appear to have some underlying logic, however, and analysis of that logic provides the optimist not only with a means of speculating about future wars, but also with an illuminating window to the inner workings of the affliction itself.

World War I was characterized by static trench warfare, with limited movement accompanied by unprecedented volumes of artillery fire. "Shell-shock", though not the neurological entity it was first assumed to be, was nevertheless not an inappropriate label for the stuporous, dazed, tremulous, confused soldiers who presented themselves to the medical system, or even for the apparently blind, deaf, or paralyzed who were brought in by their fellows. Shell shock, however, had long since been abandoned for the more sophisticated "psychoneurosis" when U.S. troops ran up against the Afriker Corps. For less sophisticated soldiers, this term translated to "psycho", and Glass (1973) suggests that this might be the reason why so many of the early psychiatric casualties of this campaign showed such dramatic and bizarre symptoms, including gross tremors, explosive startle reactions, tearing at the ground, freezing into statue-like catatonia, or withdrawal into childlike retardation or excitement. Unlike the previous world war, this war did not bog down into fixed lines but became a war of movement, with distant objectives to be achieved, mainly by foot, with required food, ammunition, and other supplies on the backs of soldiers. Very soon, as we have seen above, "exhausted" became the best descriptor of the average soldier (Bill Mauldin's Willie and Joe convey this better than thousands of words), and "exhaustion" or "combat fatigue" became the best description of the psychiatric casualties of both the Mediterranean and Pacific theatres. This is not to say that these men were merely tired or that their officers, line and medical, had any difficulty distinguishing "fatigued" from "combat-fatigued" soldiers, for in addition to a near universal tiredness, combat fatigue cases showed a variety of additional symptoms. These fell into four categories, according to Swank (1949), and, according to both Swank and to Bartemeier et al. (1946), typically appeared at different points in the evolution and treatment of the disorder.

Symptoms of *emotional tension*, especially irritability and, ironically, difficulty in sleeping, were almost always the first symptoms of breakdown. Tremulousness and exaggerated startle reactions were also common, often accompanied by feelings of inadequacy and insecurity. Although an unusually traumatic incident occasionally escalated the severity of these symptoms sufficiently for the soldier to become ineffective, more often he did not become a casualty until a second class of symptoms appeared: *disturbances of grasp or mentation*. This set of symptoms, which often replaced those of emotional tension, included general retardation, manifested by slow responses to questioning and difficulty in doing familiar everyday acts. Memory defects were often present, to the extent that the man could not be counted on to carry out simple orders, and all spontaneity of thought and action disappeared. Perhaps most striking, under the circumstances, was an apparent apathy or "affective flattening," with loss of interest in comrades, military activity, food, even letters from home, and a tendency to seclusion. For the "old sergeant" and other veterans for whom loss of a close comrade was the "last straw," deep depression was the most common and most apparent symptom, a symptom or set of symptoms which Bartemeier et al. (1946) assert is characteristic of the "exhaustion center stage" as well, no matter what the precipitating incident or experiences of the soldier. That is, cases that did not respond to treatment at the battalion aid station or division clearing station now found themselves, one to four days out of combat, separated from their unit and friends, feeling ashamed of being unable to "stick it out" with them. If they had not appeared already, the third class of symptoms typically became prominent at this point as well.

Somatic symptoms included headache, faintness or lightheadedness, backache, gastric distress, polyuria, dyspnea, and heart palpitations. Swank (1949) reports that headache, gastric distress, or backache was the initial somatic symptom in practically every case he studied, and by far the most common overall. Hospitalization seemed to fixate these symptoms, and vague, undifferentiated complaints about "not feeling well" became clearer and more clinical "symptoms." Swank (1949) even describes a group of cases who showed higher incidence of somatic symptoms after three to four months in a hastily formed quartermaster company than when they had been initially removed from their combat jobs.

The most commonly advanced explanations of such "paradoxical" findings rely on the concepts of secondary gain and survivor guilt. Hospitalization, for whatever reason, removed a combat soldier from the field of greatest danger. For the mainly ambulatory NP patient, or the patient recovering from injury, surgery, or disease, remaining in this sheltered status represented a considerable advantage over the stress and strain of active duty. Although medical officers appreciated that many of the symptoms and complaints they addressed were "functional" in nature, they saw no alternative to thorough investigation, which required longer hospitalization and greater gain for the patient. Continued hospitalization required continuing symptoms, however— and symptoms of the proper type. Grinker and Spiegel (1945), for example, point out that "psychoneurosis" was not sufficient reason for grounding flying personnel, although a host of minor somatic diseases did so. "No pain, no gain" was the rule. "Pain, therefore gain" was the result.

Hospitalization has consequences beyond removing the soldier from a stressful situation, especially for the psychiatric casualty, who as we have seen above is often already beginning to question his self-worth. From the moment his leaders confirm that he is no longer an effective and valued member of their unit, he is given a new role to play—a passive, ineffective "patient." Although he is now physically safer, he has left his friends, and although he may be in the medical system, he has no wounds and it is a psychiatrist who is treating him no matter what the diagnosis. Worse, he can watch the inflow of seriously wounded comrades with whom he can contrast his own disability. In short, preservation of his own self-image demands more medical symptoms, or a larger role for those that are present.

A similar explanation can be offered for the final category of symptoms, the hysterical or *conversion* reactions. Far less common than in World War I, when the notion that "every man had his breaking point" had yet to be recognized, conversion reactions are the dramatic cases of blindness, deafness, mutism, or paralysis without an organic basis. We would suggest that this decline took place because such extreme reactions were no longer necessary to communicate inability to function in battle. The observation that such reactions appeared to be more common among German prisoner of war psychiatric patients (Swank, 1949; Appel, 1966) is consistent with this interpretation, because the Wehrmacht did not permit psychiatric diagnoses or acknowledge that any incapacity to perform in combat not stemming from obvious injury or disease was a matter for medical attention. In a similar vein, Appel (1966) noted that among American soldiers conversion reactions seemed more likely among elite units like the airborne, who might be expected to resist even "exhaustion" or "combat fatigue" as insufficiently manly exits from combat.

Despite the widely varied and constantly changing symptoms they saw, World War II psychiatrists perhaps altered their conception of psychiatric casualties most profoundly as a result of the undeniable emergence of *group dynamics* as the key determinant of the "breaking point." By this we mean to point to the recognition of the sustaining influence of the small combat group, in what was then termed "group identification," "group cohesiveness," or "group bonds." Present-day writers might instead use the term "social support" and have no difficulty assigning it an important place in mental health, but the notion that the absence or inadequacy of these sustaining relationships was the major determinant of psychiatric breakdown in battle was quite foreign to psychiatry in the 1940s. By the end of the war, however, it was clear that differences in the incidence of psychiatric disorders in various units had more to do with characteristics of the unit than with characteristics of the casualties themselves. As Weinstein (1947) later put it:

The main characteristic of the soldier with a combat-induced neurosis is that he has become a frightened, lonely, helpless person whose interpersonal relationships have been disrupted. . . . He had lost the feeling that he was part of a powerful group and had become instead a lonely and frightened person whose efforts to protect himself were doomed to failure (p. 307).

Bartemeier et al. (1946) point to the nature of precipitating incidents as confirmation of the critical importance of group bonds, or "the soldier's position in the constellation of his social group, the combat team" (p. 369). They point out that reviewing the details of individual cases reveals that the soldier was often able to carry on in combat for considerable time, under conditions of extreme danger and discomfort. Finally, an event took place which the soldier's defenses at last could not encompass. The actual events varied tremendously, ranging from things as simple as a friendly gesture from the enemy or an unexpected change in orders to the death of a leader or buddy. The common denominator of these precipitating events, according to Bartemeier et al.

(1946), was not so much that they were the last straw in any quantitative sense, but rather that they involved a sudden change in the basic pattern of the soldier-group relationship. This might be an actual change in the structure of the group or something affecting the individual directly, and subsequently his relationship to the group. In either case he lost his place as a member of the team; alone now, he was overwhelmed and became disorganized. Bartemeier et al. (1946) acknowledge that individualistic American civilian psychiatrists and other physicians of that era might have difficulty allotting so large a role to the group, but argue that this is because nowhere in civilian life is the group of such major and crucial importance in the life of the individual as it is for the soldier in combat.

Psychiatrists, even psychoanalysts, who served in the military's forward treatment echelons had no difficulty with the central role of the group. Grinker and Spiegel (1945) provide eloquent testimony from their experiences with the army air forces. "Combat units of the Air Forces," they write, "are unique associations of men. . . . with all other emotional attitudes becoming secondary to the need to be strong and protected, and united against the enemy" (p. 21). Even such powerful forces such as anti-semitism and anti-catholicism, they say, are not likely to interfere with the camaraderie of a combat crew, though lack of experience and inability to identify with a group are serious risk factors for the combat solider. Weinberg (1946), Weinstein (1947, 1973), and Spiegel (1973) all point out the consequences of such group identification: the men were motivated to fight not by ideology or hate, but by regard for their comrades, respect for their leaders, concern for their own reputation with both, and an urge to contribute to the success of the group. In return, the group provided structure and meaning to an otherwise alien existence, a haven from an impersonal process apparently intent on grinding the life from all involved. S. L. A. Marshall, the army's premier combat historian, may have provided the clearest statement of this notion in summarizing his observations in four wars (1978): "I hold it to be one of the simplest truths of war that the thing which enables an infantry soldier to keep going with his weapon is the near presence or presumed presence of a comrade" (p. 42).

With the general acceptance of this view, the American Army had come full circle, from viewing psychiatric casualties as unfortunate aberrations best explained by their own weakness and an unusually stressful incident, to seeing "battle fatigue" as a normal and natural consequence of extended combat, staved off by some better than by others only by virtue of supportive relationships to their unit and leaders.

Treatment

As we have pointed out above, a heavy initial reliance on screening left the U.S. Army singularly unprepared to implement Salmon's World War I treatment principles of immediacy, proximity, and expectancy. Not only was the Medical Department not equipped doctrinally, but also organizationally. The lack of psychiatrists and even positions for psychiatrists forward of theatre and corps levels prevented rapid application of Salmon's principles even when they were recognized as still relevant. Organized psychiatric effort was nonexistent in the early North African operations, but psychiatry in the Mediterranean theatre finally evolved a three-echelon system much like that of World War I: division level, supported by a second echelon of special psychiatric facilities at field army level and a third echelon of base hospitals well out of the combat area. Treatment varied considerably across echelons, in part because of variations in the facilities, equipment and manpower available, and in part because the hierarchical nature of the system left the second and third echelons only patients who had failed to improve with treatment at the lower echelons.

For most combat soldiers, treatment began at the battalion aid stations, where young physicians and enlisted corpsmen without formal training in psychiatry had to decide whether to give him some hot food and hold him for a few hours or overnight, send him on to the division clearing station, or return him to the front with a pat on the back (or lower). No records were kept at the battalion aid station level, but Brill (1966) reports that many division surgeons and medical officers estimated that 40 to 50 percent of all NP casualties were returned to duty in a relatively short time by the battalion aid station. In most cases this was accomplished with a regimen of rest, replenishment, and reassurance. Perhaps the unique contribution of World War II to this twenty-five-year old prescription was the frequent use of sedatives (sodium amytal or other barbiturates) to force rest on those too anxious to fall asleep. Treatment at division clearing stations was similar in nature, but casualties could be held three to four days here if necessary. It was often easier to provide hot food and showers, fluids, and rest here, but more specific treatment was generally available only when a patient was evacuated to an "exhaustion center" or still further to a general hospital or special psychiatric hospital outside the combat zone. Treatments at these sites included individual and group talk therapy focused on the immediate past (battle) and the immediate future (return to battle). The distant past, relations within one's family, and distant future goals got little attention. The object instead was to get the patient to verbalize the horror and terror of battle and come to grips with such normal powerful emotions as grief, guilt, remorse, and fear.

As was the case with discharge and admission statistics, return-to-duty rates varied wildly between facilities, over time, and as a function of command policy. Early in the Tunisia Campaign, when all psychiatric casualties were evacuated hundreds of miles to hospitals in Algiers, Oran, and Casablanca, only 3 percent returned to combat duty. With the establishment of forward treatment facilities and policies, this figure grew to 50 to 70 percent (Wiltse, 1965).

A similar evolution took place in the Sicilian and Italian Campaigns: the leading forces were "tooth" heavy, and hence evacuated all casualties, including psychiatric, far to the rear, resulting in extremely low return rates. Drayer and Glass (1973) note that the ninety-mile evacuation across the water from Sicily to Bizerte in North Africa seemed to be critical in causing fixation of symptoms and in negating any motivation to rejoin the combat unit. Later, when battle conditions had stabilized enough to establish evacuation hospitals in Sicily, approximately 50 percent of "exhaustion" cases were returned to duty. A similar rate was reported to Kaufman and Beaton (1973) for the South Pacific during 1944, and a slightly higher rate (65 percent) for the Seventh Army in Europe over the final nine months of the war. It should be noted, however, that return rates varied from 33 to 89 percent across the twelve divisions comprising the Seventh Army (Thompson, Talkington, and Ludwig, 1973), and that division clearing stations generally had return rates half again as high as army-level hospitals. Direct comparison of divisions or of clearing stations and hospitals is fraught with danger, for the ability to return patients is not independent of either incidence or admissions criteria, and hospital psychiatrists as a general rule attempted treatment only on patients whom a clearing station had already failed to return to duty. Nevertheless, the figures do confirm that psychiatric casualties are eminently treatable and constitute a valuable source of manpower within the combat theatre.

A final and perhaps most important contribution of World War II psychiatrists in the area of treatment stemmed from their recognition, detailed above, of the crucial importance of group identification as a sustaining mechanism for the combat soldier. With this recognition it became obvious why Salmon's brief, simple, forward treatment principles worked as well as they did. For the patient, caught like all soldiers in a struggle between conflicting desires to return to the group which has become the center of his existence and to flee forever this terrifying battlezone, brief treatment close to the lines succeeds because time and distance have not yet eroded the bonds between soldier and unit. Reassurance and persuasion directly aimed at returning the soldier to his unit emphasize these bonds and restore an endangered equilibrum. Evacuation to a comfortable hospital far in the near, on the other hand, for treatment by frequently guilt-ridden personnel not fully convinced of their patients' need to return to the battle, tips this delicate balance to the side of self-preservation. The accompanying feelings of failure and loss of self-esteem promote continued or elaborated symptomatology, however, a consequence not readily amenable to attempts to alter or reorganize the personality with uncovering depth techniques (Spiegel, 1944, Glass, 1954; Coleman, 1973).

POST-WORLD WAR II

In October 1945, after a lengthy series of consultations with many military and civilian psychiatrists, the army surgeon general issued a revised nomenclature system reflecting many of the lessons learned during the war. Its central feature was the addition of two new diagnostic categories: transient personality reactions and immaturity reactions. The first included "all emotional reaction to acute and special stress" under "combat exhaustion" or, for disorders resulting from unusual or overwhelming stress under noncombat conditions, "acute situational maladjustments." Neurotic-type reactions to routine military stress, particularly if marked by helplessness, passive obstructionism, or aggressive outbursts, were to be classified as "immaturity reactions." These new diagnoses effectively took the military psychiatrist off the horns of his "psychoneurosis" or "normal" dilemma. Shortly afterwards, the American Psychiatric Association included their essential features in a revision of its official diagnostic nomenclature.

KOREA

The outbreak of hostilities in Korea in June 1950 found many of the army's World War II psychiatrists still in uniform, and most of their knowledge and experience was institutionalized in regulations, training manuals, and other military publications. As a result, division psychiatry became operational within two months of the onset of fighting. By October 1950, the three-echelon system of World War II combat psychiatry had been established, and the largely successful results of the latter half of World War II were achieved once more (Marren, 1956). Several aspects of our Korean War experience were novel enough to merit further comment, however.

The most prominent of these Korean War "novelties" was something called "*short-termer's syndrome*" (Glass, 1953) or "rotation anxiety" (Norbury, 1953), which ironically emerged as a direct result of the armed forces' well-intentioned attempts to ward off "combat fatigue" in general and "Old Sergeant's Syndrome" in particular. Taking as a given the World War II phrase "every man has his breaking point," a nine-month rotation policy was established in Korea, to insure that honorable relief from battle could be obtained by a means other than by death, wounds, or psychiatric dysfunction. The general consensus (Marren, 1956; Glass, 1953) is that the lower admissions, evacuation, and discharge rates of Korea, relative to World War II, were at least in part attributable to this innovation, but there was a price paid. One of the most obvious effects of rotation was the disruption of the sustaining power of group identification that occurred when a soldier began to approach the end of his tour. Combat now became an individual struggle, as the short-termer, who had previously borne the usual discomfort and dangers of battle, disengaged himself from his buddies. The subsequent rise in anxiety sometimes became disabling, aided by the ubiquitous stories of some unfortunate killed the day before he was scheduled to rotate. Everyone understood the syndrome as a normal phenomenon, and the short-termer was often spontaneously protected by the other men of his unit (no doubt with a view toward similar treatment in the future), who saw to it that he spent his final days in relatively safe assignments or, if symptoms were too severe, got him medically evacuated. Even in the latter case however, the soldier would nearly always simply be held until normal rotation rather than be evacuated through medical channels. Glass (1953) suggests that the removal of entire combat units, or at least their older or original members, would perhaps be the most effective form of rotation despite the increased logistical burden it would impose. Lavin (1953) would appear to agree, as he reports very favorable results (decreased NP cases, accidental injuries, sick call attendance, and disciplinary problems) from a program of regularly rotating companies and battalions out of the line for a few days' rest and relaxation which was initiated in his division.

The signing of an armistice in Korea in July 1953 resulted in quite a different state of affairs for the troops involved than the November 1918 armistice or the surrender of Germany and Japan in 1945. The stalemate conceded by the signature of the Korean armistice necessitated the maintenance of large, fully armed, constantly alert forces by both sides, trained, equipped, and poised to strike on a moment's notice. As a result, American troops, despite relief from the obvious stresses of battle, continued to suffer psychiatric casualties, at a rate not markedly less than the rates characteristic of the combat years. These cases were obviously not combat fatigue in the absence of combat, but they might be called combat zone fatigue. Harris (1954) points out the need to distinguish actual fighting and life in the combat zone, for he says these two situations spawn two broad types of psychiatric problems, one more dramatic but well defined in onset and etiology, and usually transient, the other less serious but more difficult to understand and eliminate. A freeze-in-place armistic like that of 1953, it might be argued, should eliminate the first of these patient groups but leave the second intact. Marren (1956) goes further, arguing that many hardships, tolerable in the heat of battle or relatively inconsequential relative to the stark terror of actual fighting, assume far greater importance in the absence of gun fire. Food, shelter, sanitation, bathing and recreational facilities, even if much improved from pre-armistice conditions, were still wretched substitutes for their stateside equivalents. Meaningless activity, or inactivity, became a burden, as did problems back home, and discipline, recognized as essential for survival in combat, now seemed arbitrary and capricious. In addition, says Marren (1956), the supportive bonds to comrades and leaders formed by sharing dull and tedious duties are only pale copies of those forged in the heat of combat. The "immaturity reactions" and "character and behavior disorders" which resulted would not be seen in such large numbers again until Richard Nixon began the withdrawal of U.S. troops from Vietnam.

Two final features of psychiatry in the Korean conflict, while not unique to that war, were underscored by their prominence there. First, the bitter winters of Korea provided a new example of a somatic psychiatric syndrome shaped by an endemic medical problem. Just as the medical officer in the South Pacific theatre of World War II was forced to decide if the weak, tremulous, sweating patient before him was a malaria victim or a psychiatric casualty, so in Korea, his counterpart was asked to make a similar decision about the patient before him complaining of pain or lack of feeling in his toes. Was this frostbite or merely cold feet? As Glass (1953) points out, the increased sympathetic stimulation resulting from a high level of anxiety may have caused excessive vasoconstriction of the extremities, but whatever the reason, an increased incidence of frostbite diagnoses was accompnied by a decrease in psychiatric cases.

Finally, and not unrelated to the frostbite/cold feet issue, the very drastic swings in the tide of battle which characterized the Korean conflict underscored the enormous influence of the combat situation on manifestations of combat ineffectiveness. In July 1950, and again in December 1950, U.S. forces were driven southward by numerically superior forces. Despite large numbers of killed, wounded, and injured, there were relatively few psychiatric casualties. On both of these occasions, medical facilities were minimal and were themselves under attack. In short, it was safer to remain with the group than risk becoming a straggler. We have already addressed this notion of gain through illness, and it also probably can account for the very small number of psychiatric casualties sustained: on patrols beyond the frontlines, despite the extremely hazardous nature of the task; among naval personnel in battle at sea; and among prisoners of war and civilian populations under bombardment (Glass, 1953, 1957; Harris, 1956).

VIETNAM

Military psychiatry, like many other aspects of the Vietnam conflict, can best be seen as composed of three distinct periods: pre-Tet, post-Tet, and postwar. Each period had its distinctive political, strategic, and tactical features, its own stressors, modes of ineffectiveness, and psychiatric response.

Reports on psychiatric support in the early years of the conflict were notable for the pride with which it was noted that diligent application of lessons learned in the World Wars and in Korea had succeeded in holding psychiatric casualties to an unprecedented low. Allerton (1969), for example, reported that over a twelve-month period in 1967–1968, divisions (with 16,000 to 17,000 men each) evacuated an average of only four patients per month. Tiffany (1967) reported the 1965–1966 NP casualty incidence as 12 per thousand, and Bourne and San (1967) noted that only 6 percent of all medical evacuations from Vietnam had been for psychiatric reasons, compared with 23 percent in World War II. All pointed out that these psychiatric admission and evacuation rates were lower than those in any previous war, and allotted much of the credit to a vigorous preventive psychiatry effort and increased psychiatric sophistication among both medical and line officers. Bourne (1969) was encouraged enough to assert that "our level of knowledge of combat psychology has now reached the point where with adequate vigilance psychiatric casualties need never again became a major cause of attrition in the United States military in a combat zone" (p. 231).

Others, including Glass (1969), Colbach and Parrish (1970), and Pettera, Johnson, and Zimmer (1969), did not contest the figures but gave much more credit to the nature of the war: intermittent fighting, secure and comfortable base camps, the relatively slight capacity of the enemy for aerial or artillery bombardment, and the one-year individualized rotation policy. Still others, for example, Jones (1967a and b), Kenny (1967), Tischler (1969), and Renner (1973), pointed out that, not only was the number of cases lower, but the nature of the psychiatric cases they were seeing was different from that of past wars. "Combat fatigue" cases were practically nonexistent, except for the very rare set-piece battle (Motis, 1968), although Jones and Johnson (1975) point out that combat soldiers presented with somatic complaints for which no organic basis could be found and suggest that physicians' reluctance to use such an unscientific and guilt-producing label as "combat fatigue" may have contributed to the very low rate of such diagnoses. Regardless of the true rate of combat fatigue, a large proportion of psychiatric admissions was from the noncombat elements of the military in Vietnam. These soldiers were seldom seen by the Medical Department until administrative or punitive measures were being considered, and most often the primary diagnosis ended up with "character and behavior disorder" (Jones, 1967a and b) or "personality disorder" (Renner, 1973). Drug abuse, excessive alcohol use, depression, and repeated disciplinary problems were the behaviors most often cited. Dowling (1967) and Tischler (1970) even relate such behaviors to the one-year rotation: an initial period producing a high incidence of sleep walking and other sleep disorders, anxiety, and somatic complaints; a middle period, in which depression and drug and alcohol abuse increased; and a terminal period, in which a short-timers' syndrome was again seen and disciplinary problems came to the fore. In short, we had held tight to the lessons of the past wars regarding combat fatigue but had failed even to notice the lessons in combat-zone fatigue which the Korean War made available.

The real significance of these "disorders of loneliness" (Jones and Johnson, 1975) was realized only after the Tet Offensive of the North Vietnamese Army and the Vietcong in 1968. These desperate efforts marked the beginning of the end of the war, although it would be five years until a peace agreement was signed. During these five years of "Vietnamization," U.S. troops were increasingly relegated to a support role, and they were characterized by nearly universally low morale, captured in the graffiti initials U.U.U.U.—the unwilling, led by the unqualified, doing the unnecessary for the ungrateful. The psychiatric admission rates in 1970 (25.1 per thousand per year) just about doubled those of 1968, despite the fact that the number of wounded in action was cut by 60 percent (Neel, 1973). Out-of-country psychiatric evacuation, which accounted for less than 5 percent of medical evacuations until the first quarter of 1971, abruptly increased by a factor of 10, and the outpatient psychiatric treatment rate doubled (Jones and Johnson, 1975). A substantial percentage of these increases was related to large-scale drug screening which began about the same time. That is, drug-dependent soldiers were being evacuated as psychiatric casualties. By all accounts, however, these constituted only a tiny portion of drug users, and the rates failed to include those whose attempts at coping led to other kinds of active or passive aggression. Racial disturbances, disciplinary infractions of all types, and attacks on superiors (fragging) grew steadily. "Search and avoid" missions were the responses of combat soldiers determined not to be the last to die in Vietnam, and resentful compliance with the letter of the law won bored, lonely, anxious, and angry support soldiers an uneasy stalemate with their leaders (Camp, 1985).

Ironically, the twelve-month rotation system which had been hailed as a major factor in reducing battle fatigue cases in the pre-Tet era now, as in Korea, appeared to be a substantial contributor to poor morale and attendant behavioral problems. First, it insured a continuing influx of new soldiers, drafted from an increasingly antiwar populace. Second, it made the war a very individualized event for most soldiers, whose only objective became reaching DEROS (Date of Expected Return from Over Seas) intact. It thus weakened or removed from the soldier the social support from his unit that sustained his predecessors. Other policies and circumstances insured that possible mitigating factors were eliminated as well. The common danger that created strong bonds in the combat units of the 1960s became less common as the United States more and more assumed an advisory and support role; the excellent mail and even telephone service that had enabled pre-Tet soldiers to derive emotional support from family and friends in the United States now often provided instead confirmation of their feelings that they were being treated unfairly; and the policy of providing "command experience" to officers by splitting their year into six months in command and six months in a staff job only made it seem more obvious that it was every man for himself. Many (e.g., Bey and Zecchinelli, 1971; Bentel, Smith, and Crim, 1971; Renner, 1973; and Ingraham, 1974) recognized drug use as a quick means of identifying with a group and gaining the interpersonal relationships the system seemed to be trying so hard to deny the soldier. The "group" thus formed seldom had any motivation to further the mission of its military unit however, and often saw its officers and NCOs (the "lifers") as its enemy instead. The net result for psychiatrists like Camp (1985) was feeling

> overwhelmed by the extensive numbers of soldiers with various manifestations of low morale (apathy, defiance, drug abuse without addiction, assaultive behavior, etc.), and an appreciation that we were relatively unable to correct these matters. . . . .The net result was that our team served a limited role, unsatisfying to these soldiers, to the commanders who referred them, and to us (p. 4).

The twelve-month rotation not only injected men into Vietnam as individual replacements (though we knew well from World War II that this maximized their vulnerability to psychological as well as physical stress), but it also extracted them individually, often depositing them on the street back in "the world" as civilians only twenty-four hours after leaving base camp. We are only now beginning to realize what a mistake this was as we continue to grapple with the Vietnam conflict's most distinctive legacy: post-traumatic stress disorder (PTSD). Described by DSM-III as a reaction to a psychologically traumatic event outside the range of normal experience, PTSD manifestations include recurrent and intrusive dreams and recollections of the experience, emotional blunting, social withdrawal, especially difficulty or reluctance in initiating or maintaining intimate relationships, and sleep disturbances. These symptoms can in turn lead to serious difficulties in readjusting to civilian life, including alcoholism, divorce, and unemployment. The distinguishing feature, however, is the persistence of the symptoms for months or years after the obvious trauma—or the emergence of symptoms only after a long delay. Estimates of the number of civilian Vietnam veterans suffering from PTSD range from 500,000 (Disabled American Veterans Association, 1980) to 1.5 million (Harris and Associates, 1980). This represents 18 to 54 percent of the 2.8 million military personnel who served in Vietnam. Although Glass (1953) mentions in passing, and Figley (1978), on the basis of questionnaire data, asserts that a significant percentage of veterans from all wars are plagued with dreams and nightmares related to their wartime experience, the relative paucity of literature on post-combat reactions among World War II and Korean veterans makes it likely that outward manifestations of discontent or maladjustment are far more common among Vietnam veterans. There is not yet enough published data to say whether PTSD is more likely among vets who served early in the war or vets who served in the 1970s, but at least some literature suggests the opposite of what we might expect by simply equating combat and trauma. Borus (1974) compared 577 soldiers who had completed Vietnam tours at the end of 1970 with 172 soldiers who had never been to Vietnam and found no significant differences in extent of maladjustment. Nace, Myers, O'Brien, and Ream (1975) examined 202 veterans who had served in Vietnam two or three years prior to the interview, in 1971 and 1972. He concluded that a full one-third of this sample showed signs of clinical depression, despite doing their Vietnam tour in a period when the trauma of combat was less probable and less frequent than in previous years. Something else must be involved.

Theories about this something else can, with a bit of oversimplification, be sorted into two types: those that point to characteristics of the soldiers themselves (e.g., Silsby and Jones, 1985; Worthington, 1977; Rosenheck, 1985; Hendin and Haas, 1984), and those that point to characteristics of the war (e.g., Defazio, 1975; Brown, 1984; Frye and Stockton, 1982; Leventman, 1978; and Lifton, 1974). As a group, the first type seems to offer some very plausible reasons why some suffer and others manage to put their tour behind them—but in most cases fail even to attempt an answer to why this particular war should produce so many more of the sufferers. Hendin and Haas (1984), for example, assert that it is "not so much what the individual experienced in Vietnam but how those events and situations were perceived, integrated, and acted upon that bears the primary relationship to postcombat response" (p. 959). Combat veterans who seemed to be dealing with postwar civilian life without any evidence of a stress disorder, we are told, in contrast to those who developed postwar stress problems, "did not perceive combat as a test of their worth as men, as an opportunity to express anger or vengeance, or as a situation in which they were powerless victims" (p. 959). Nowhere do the authors explicitly tell the reader why we might expect so many Vietnam veterans to fall in the second group.

Theories of the second sort, on the other hand, focus explicitly on this question. Defazio (1975), for example, blames the combination of a number of features of the war which he feels distinguishes it from previous wars (clandestine operations by both sides, an indigenous revolutionary army, an alien culture, the youth of our army relative to that of past wars, moral doubts about the justifiability of the war, and the public's hostility toward veterans). Other writers have compiled slightly different lists, but all assign significant weight to public antipathy to veterans. Figley (1979) perhaps puts it best in chastening his fellow psychologists about "confusing the warrior with the war" (p. 2). Empirical surveys of both soldiers (Frye and Stockton, 1982) and Veterans Administration mental health professionals (Keane and Fairbank, 1983) have repeatedly identified social support *upon return* from Vietnam as a critical factor in the development of PTSD, often considering it more critical than the intensity of combat experienced or the social support received while in Vietnam (Stretch, 1985). The combination of rapid return of individual soldiers to the United States and civilian life with indifference, fear, or even hostility of the civilian populace apparently prevented many veterans from "working through" their experiences and attaining the sense of closure possible for the vast majority of veterans of past wars who came home in units on troopships to a supportive, if not hero-worshipping, community (Brown, 1984; Egendorf, Kadushin, Laufer, Rothbart, and Sloan, 1981; and Leventman, 1978).

Lifton (1974) theorizes that the combat veteran of any war is faced with the task of attenuating indelible images of death and suffering, the anxiety and guilt that accompany them, and the social distancing and emotional blunting that have served as his defenses. This task is greatly dependent on finding meaning and justification for his fighting, killing, and even surviving. In the normal course of events, this search is aided by the assurances of family, friends, and community that his sacrifices are appreciated and justified by the importance for all of them of what he has accomplished. In the case of Vietnam, the combat veteran has all too often been able to find these assurances only among his fellow vets. The difficulties with delayed and chronic stress reactions (see Belenky in Chapter 5 of this volume) which Israel is now experiencing among veterans of their first unpopular war, the Lebanon incursion, provide a validation of this view which has direct implications for rotation and discharge policy. In particular, it would seem prudent to require all personnel departing a combat theatre to undergo a period of debriefing and decompression in the presence of fellow veterans, encouraging them to work through their experiences before returning home. Psychiatric casualties delayed are psychiatric casualties nonetheless.

CONCLUSION

Twentieth-century warfare is distinguished by its intensity and ferocity. Once the battle is joined, individual soldiers can expect neither escape nor respite. To paraphrase Grinker and Spiegel (1945), the result is a fragile equilibrium constantly threatened by situations in which the soldier faces the choice of saving his own life, perhaps to fight again but haunted by guilt, or of risking it for comrades and perhaps dying a hero's death without in the least desiring to be a hero. The vast majority of soldiers reject the easy escapes from the dilemma, surrender, desertion, and self-inflicted wounds or "accidents," but this leaves only wounding, capture, or death.

Unable and unwilling to make the rational response of fleeing for their lives, soldiers have little choice but to endure as best they can for as long as they can. There are limits, however, and for each soldier there exists a breaking point. The key concept in current American doctrine is that individual breakdown in combat is unfortunate but normal. This has been an exceedingly difficult lesson for Americans to learn. General Patton's slapping incident is only the most notorious example of the pervasive American cultural attitude that holds breakdown in combat as prima facie evidence of cowardice and moral turpitude. Despite the overwhelming evidence to the contrary, most Americans, in and out of uniform, firmly believe it is within the army's power to eliminate the unit before they ever enter service.

Reflecting on their experiences in World War II, Bartemeier and his associates (1946) observed that military psychiatry is concerned with treating normal reactions to abnormal environments, whereas civilian psychiatry focuses on treating abnormal reactions to normal environments. The tasks of army mental health professionals are to delay breakdown by preventive means, to stem contagion, and to provide rest and encouragement to those who have exceeded their limits.

Prevention entails tangling with another American sacred cow, belief in the primacy of the individual. The lesson from the American experience is that without the military group, the individual is quickly lost. Hilmar (1965) phrases it nicely:

Military life is essentially group life; the individual in the armed forces finds himself in enforced, intimate association with others during virtually all phases of his service. With rare exceptions he trains in a group, works in a group, fights in a group, sleeps and eats in a group, and more often than not, spends his leisure time as a member of a group. Furthermore, during wartime especially, all these activities tend to be conducted within the confines of the same group. In situations of great stress or dire peril the individual's survival or the successful accomplishment of the military mission or both are likely to depend largely upon the pattern of interpersonal relationship within the small groups involved (p. 311).

The American attachment to notions of rugged individualism clouds the judgment of military commanders and mental health professional alike. Unlike other contemporary and ancient armies, Americans have been content to accept small group solidarity as a desirable byproduct rather than as a first principle of sound military organization. Thus, twenty-five years after World War II the Americans were still training soldiers as individuals, sending them to their units as individuals, rotating them out as individuals, and wondering why there seemed such a high prevalence of individual dysfunction. Perhaps with more careful selection? The lessons remain difficult to master because they are so un-American.

Yet they must be mastered. The ecology of the battlefield continues to change in response to new technology, ideology, and scientific understanding. The trenches of France were not the deserts of Africa, were not the jungles of the Pacific, were not the mountains of Korea, were not the paddies of Vietnam. The presenting symptoms of the combat stress casualties were not the same either. What will be a normal reaction will depend on what defines an abnormal environment. The lethality of modern weapons mandates even greater dispersion of troops on an already terrifying and painfully lonely battlefield. The prospects of fighting in cities, in chemical protective gear with limited auditory and visual contact with buddies, in a nuclear environment, or in an uncertain political climate will continue to define acceptable responses when soldiers' spirits break and they conclude consciously or unconsciously, as their fathers, grandfathers, and great grandfathers before them, "Enough is enough, I can endure no more."

Will Americans be prepared for the next act of what seems a continuing tragedy? There is reason to hope so. Since 1981 the American Army has moved toward a unit replacement system whereby soldiers are trained together for an entire three-year enlistment. Combat team solidarity or cohesion is now an explicit goal of army reorganization efforts. Also encouraging is the provision of additional mental health personnel in the medical support element of the newly configured combat divisions. Furthermore, issues of combat stress are being addressed in more and more army schools, and a pocket card has been prepared to get the message to private soldiers and their sergeants.

Although there is reason to believe that Americans are better prepared than at any time in their history, there is no cause for complacency. It is possible the next war will be very short; the first battles will be decisive; and they are likely to generate significant combat stress casualties. There are very few mental health professionals in uniform with experience in a combat army in the field. The problems of implementating rapid treatment close to the firing will be formidable on the modern mobile battlefield. The frictions of war first described by Clausewitz remain in force: in war little goes according to plan; the most elementary fact is that America will see battle stress casualties in the next war; how many, what symptoms, what treatment, and with what results remain unknown and unknowable. Whatever optimism is warranted must be tempered with extreme caution. The problem of battle stress has been "solved" too many times this century, only to reappear where and when least expected.

REFERENCES

Allerton, William S. (1969). Army psychiatry in Viet Nam. In P. G. Bourne (ed.), *The psychology and physiology of stress*. New York: Academic Press, pp. 2–17.

Appel, J. W. (1966). Preventive psychiatry. In R. L. Bernucci and A. J. Glass (eds.), *Neuropsychiatry in World War II: Vol. 1. Zone of the interior*. Washington, D.C.: U.S. Government Printing Office, pp. 373–415.

Appel, J. W. and Beebe, G. W. (1946). Preventive psychiatry: an epidemiological approach. *Journal of the American Medical Association*, *131* (18), 1469–1475.

Armstrong, H. G. (1939). *Principles and practice of aviation medicine*. Baltimore: Williams & Wilkins Co.

Bailey, P., Williams, F. E., and Koroma, P. O. (1929). *The Medical Department of the United States Army in the World War. Vol 10, Neuropsychiatry*. Washington, D.C.: U.S. Government Printing Office.

Bartemeier, L. H., Kubie, L. S., Menninger, K. A., Romano, J., and Whitehorn, J. C. (1946). Combat exhaustion. *Journal of Nervous and Mental Disease*, *104*, 358–389, 489–525.

Beebe, G. W., and Appel, J. W. (1958). *Variation in psychological tolerance to ground combat in World War II* (Contract DA-49-007-MD-172). Washington, D.C.: Medical Research and Development Board, Office of the Surgeon General, Department of the Army. (Cited in Appel, 1966.)

Bentel, D., Smith, D., and Crim, D. (1971). Drug abuse in combat: the crisis of drugs and addiction among American troops in Vietnam. *Journal of Psychedelic Drugs*, *4*, 23–30.

Bey, D., and Zecchinelli, V. (1971). Marijuana as a coping device in Vietnam. *Military Medicine*, *136*, 448–450.
Borus, J. (1974). Incidence of maladjustment in Vietnam returnees. *Archives of General Psychiatry*, *30*, 554–557.
Bourne, P. G. (1969). Military psychiatry and the Viet Nam war in perspective. In P. G. Bourne, (ed.), *The psychology and physiology of stress*. New York: Academic Press, pp. 219–236.
Bourne, P. G. (1970). *Men, stress and Vietnam*. Boston: Little, Brown & Co.
Bourne, P. G., and San, N. D. (1967). A comparative study of neuropsychiatric casualties in the United States Army and the Army of the Republic of Vietnam. *Military Medicine*, *132*, 904–909.
Braatz, G. A., Lumry, G. K., and Wright, M. S. (1971). The young veteran as a psychiatric patient in three eras of conflict. *Military Medicine*, *136*, 455–457.
Brill, N. Q. (1966). Hospitalization and disposition. In R. L. Bernucci and A. J. Glass (eds.), *Neuropsychiatry in World War II: Vol. 1. Zone of the interior*. Washington, D.C.: U.S. Government Printing Office, pp. 195–253.
Brown, P. (1984). Legacies of a war: treatment considerations with Vietnam veterans and their families. *Social Work*, *29*, 372–378.
Camp, N. M. (1985). Dysfunction and demoralization of U.S. forces in the Vietnam conflict phasedown, Parts I and II. Unpublished manuscript. Washington, D.C.: Walter Reed Army Institute of Research.
Churchill, W. S. (1933). *Marlborough, his life and times*. London: Leo Cooper.
Colbach, E., and Parrish, M. (1970). Army mental health activities in Vietnam: (1965–1970). *Bulletin of the Menninger Clinic*, *31*, 333–342.
Coleman, J. V. (1973). Division psychiatry in the Southwest Pacific area. In W. S. Mullens, and A. J. Glass (eds.), *Neuropsychiatry in World War II: Vol. 2. Overseas Theatres*. Washington, D.C.: U.S. Government Printing Office, pp. 623–637.
Defazio, V. J. (1975). The Vietnam era veteran: psychological problems. *Journal of Contemporary Psychotherapy*, *7*, 9–15.
Deutsch, A. (1944). Military psychiatry: the Civil War, 1861–1865. In American Psychiatric Association (ed.), *One hundred years of American psychiatry: 1844–1944*. New York: Columbia University Press, pp. 367–384.
Disabled American Veterans Association (1980). *Forgotten Warriors: America's Vietnam era veterans*. Washington, D.C.: Author.
Dowling, J. (1967). Psychologic aspects of the year in Vietnam. *U.S. Army of Vietnam Medical Bulletin*, *3*, (May-June), 45–48.
Drayer, C. S., and Glass, A. J. (1973). Introduction. In W. S. Mullens and A. J. Glass (eds.), *Neuropsychiatry in World War II: Vol. 2. Overseas*

Theaters. Washington, D.C.: U.S. Government Printing Office, pp. 1–23.

Egendorf, A., Kadushin, C., Laufer, R., Rothbart, G., and Sloan, L. (1981). *Legacies of Vietnam: comparative adjustment of veterans and their peers.* New York: Center For Policy Research.

Figley, C. R. (1978). Psychological adjustment among Vietnam veterans: an overview of the research. In C. R. Figley (ed.), *Stress disorders among Vietnam veterans.* New York: Brunner-Mazel.

Figley, C. R. (1978). Symptoms of delayed combat stress among college sample of Vietnam veterans. *Military Medicine, 143,* 107–110.

Figley, C. R. (1979). Confusing the warrior with the war. *APA Monitor,* April, 2.

Frye, J., and Stockton, R. (1982). Discriminant analysis of post-traumatic stress disorder among a group of Vietnam veterans. *American Journal of Psychiatry, 139,* 52–56.

Ginzberg, E., (1959). *The lost divisions.* New York: Columbia University Press.

Glass, A. J. (1953). Psychiatry in the Korean campaign. A historical review. *U.S. Armed Forces Medical Journal, 4* (11), 1563–1583.

Glass, A. J. (1954). Psychotherapy in the combat zone. *American Journal of Psychiatry, 110* (10), 725–731.

Glass, A. J. (1957). *Observations upon the epidemiology of mental illness in troops during warfare.* Symposium on Preventive and Social Psychiatry. Washington, D.C.: Walter Reed Army Institute of Research.

Glass, A. J. (1966). Lessons learned. In R. L. Bernucci and A. J. Glass (eds.), *Neuropsychiatry in World War II: Vol. 1. Zone of the interior.* Washington, D.C.: U.S. Government Printing Office, pp. 735–759.

Glass, A. J. (1969). Introduction. In P. G. Bourne (ed.), *The psychology and physiology of stress.* New York: Academic Press, pp. xiii–xxv

Glass, A. J. (1973). Lessons learned. In W. S. Mullens and A. J. Glass (eds.), *Neuropsychiatry in World War II: Vol. 2. Overseas theaters.* Washington, D.C.: U.S. Government Printing Office, pp. 989–1027.

Glass, A. J., and Drayer, C. S. (1973). Italian campaign (1 March 1944-2 May 1945), Psychiatry established at division level. In W. S. Mullens and A. J. Glass (eds.), *Neuropsychiatry in World War II: Vol. 2. Overseas theaters.* Washington, D.C.: U.S. Government Printing Office, pp. 989–1027.

Grinker, R. R., and Spiegel, J. P. (1945). *Men under stress.* New York: McGraw-Hill.

Harris, F. G. (1954). Some comments on the differential diagnosis and treatment of psychiatric breakdowns in Korea. Abstract of the presentation given to the Course on Recent Advances in Medicine and Surgery,

Army Medical Service Graduate School, Walter Reed Army Medical Center, Washington, D.C.

Harris, F. G. (1956). Experiences in the study of combat in the Korean theater. II. Comments on a concept of psychiatry for a combat zone. (WRAIR Research Report 165-66.) Washington, D.C.: Walter Reed Army Institute of Research.

Harris, L., and Associates. (1980). *Myths and realities: a study of attitudes toward Vietnam era veterans.* U.S. Senate Committee on Veterans Affairs, Print No 29. Washington, D.C.: U.S. Government Printing Office.

Hausman, W., and Rioch, D. Mck. (1967). A prototype of social and preventive psychiatry in the United States. *Archives of General Psychiatry, 16,* 727–739.

Hendin, H., and Haas, A. (1984). Combat adaptation of Vietnam veterans without posttraumatic stress disorders. *American Journal of Psychiatry, 141,* 956–960.

Hilmar, N. A. (1965). The dynamics of military group behavior. In C. H. Coates and R. J. Pelligrin (eds.), *Military sociology: a study of American military institutions in military life.* Baltimore, Md.: Social Science Press, Ch. 13.

Ingraham, L. (1974). The Nam and the world: heroin use by U.S. Army men in Vietnam. *Psychiatry, 37,* 114–128.

Jones, F. D. (1967a). Viet duty causes varied "psychoses." *U.S. Medicine,* 2–3.

Jones, F. D. (1967b). Experiences of a division psychiatrist in Vietnam. *Military Medicine, 132,* 1003–1008.

Jones, F. D., and Johnson, A. W. (1975). Medical and psychiatric treatment policy and practice in Vietnam. *Journal of Social Issues, 31* (4), 49–65.

Kaufman, M. R., and Beaton, L. E. (1973). South Pacific area. In W. S. Mullens and A. J. Glass, (eds.), *Neuropsychiatry in World War II: Vol. 2. Overseas theaters.* Washington, D.C.: U.S. Government Printing Office, pp. 429–472.

Keane, T., and Fairbank, J. (1983). Survey analysis of combat-related stress disorders in Vietnam veterans. *American Journal of Psychiatry, 140,* pp. 212–218.

Kenny, W. F. (1967). Psychiatric disorders among support personnel. *USARV Medical Bulletin,* 34–37.

Levin, R. J. (1953). Division psychiatry. *U.S. Army Medical Bulletin Far East,* 137–140.

Leventman, S. (1978). Epilogue: social and historical perspectives on the

Vietnam veterans. In C. R. Figley (ed.), *Stress disorders among Vietnam veterans*. New York: Brunner-Mazel, pp. 291-296.

Lifton, R. (1974). Death imprints on youth in Vietnam. *Journal of Clinical Child Psychology, 3*, 47-49.

Marren, J. J. (1956). Psychiatric problems in troops in Korea during and following combat. *U.S. Armed Forces Medical Journal, 7* (5), 715-726.

Marshall, S. L. A. (1978). *Men against fire.* Gloucester, Mass.: Peter Smith.

Motis, G. (1968). Psychiatry at the battle of Dak To. *U.S. Army Vietnam Medical Bulletin*, February, 27-30.

Nace, E., Meyers, A., O'Brien, C., and Ream, N. (1975). Depression in veterans two years after Vietnam. Unpublished manuscript.

Neel, S. (1973). *Medical support of the U.S. Army in Vietnam 1965-1970.* Washington, D.C.: U.S. Department of the Army.

Norbury, F. B. (1953). Psychiatric admissions in a combat division in 1952. *U.S. Army Medical Bulletin Far East*, 130-133.

Pettera, R. L., Johnson, B. M., and Zimmer, R. (1969). Psychiatric management of combat reactions with emphasis on a reaction unique to Vietnam. *Military Medicine, 134*, 673-678.

Renner, J. A. (1973). The changing patterns of psychiatric problems in Vietnam. *Comprehensive Psychiatry, 14* (2), 169-181.

Richardson, F. M. (1978). *Fighting spirit.* London: Leo Cooper.

Rosenheck, R. (1985). Malignant post-Vietnam stress syndrome. *American Journal of Orthopsychiatry, 55*, 166-176.

Salmon, T. W., and Fenton, N. (1929). Neuropsychiatry in the American Expeditionary Forces. In P. Bailey, F. E. Williams, and P. O. Komora (eds.), *The Medical Department of the United States Army in the World War Vol 10. Neuropsychiatry.* Washington, D.C.: U.S. Government Printing Office.

Silsby, H. D., and Jones, F. D. (1985). The etiologies of Vietnam post-traumatic stress syndrome. *Military Medicine, 150*, 6-7.

Spiegel, H. X. (1944). Psychiatric observations in the Tunisian campaign. *American Journal of Orthopsychiatry*, 381-385.

Spiegel, H. X. (1973). Psychiatry with an infantry battalion in North Africa. In W. S. Mullens and A. J. Glass (eds.), *Neuropsychiatry in World War II. Vol. II: Overseas theaters.* Washington, D.C.: U.S. Government Printing Office, pp. 111-126.

Stretch, R. A. (1985). Post-traumatic stress disorder among Vietnam and Vietnam-era veterans. In C. R. Figley (ed.), *Trauma and its wake: the study and treatment of post-traumatic stress disorder.* New York: Brunner-Mazel.

Swank, R. L., and Marchand, W. E. (1946). Combat neuroses: development

of combat exhaustion. *Archives of Neurology and Psychology, 55*, 236–247.
Swank, R. L. Combat exhaustion. (1949). *Journal of Nervous and Mental Disease, 109* (6), 475–508.
Thompson, L. J., Talkington, P. X., and Ludwig, A. O. (1973). Neuropsychiatry at army and division levels. In W. S. Mullens and A. J. Glass (eds.), *Neuropsychiatry in World War II. Vol. 2: Overseas theaters.* Washington, D.C.: U.S. Government Printing Office, pp. 275–374.
Tiffany, W. J., Jr. (1967). The mental health of army troops in Viet Nam. *American Journal of Psychiatry, 123* (12), 1585–1586.
Tischler, G. L. (1969). Patterns of psychiatric attrition and of behavior in a combat zone. In P. Bourne (ed.), *The psychology and physiology of stress.* New York: Academic Press, pp. 19–44.
Weinberg, S. K. (1946). The combat neuroses. *American Journal of Sociology, 51*, 465–478.
Weinstein, E. A. (1947). The function of interpersonal relations in the neurosis of combat. *Psychiatry, 10*, 307-314.
Weinstein, E. A. (1973). The Fifth U.S. Army Neuropsychiatric Center—'601 st.' In W. S. Mullens and A. J. Glass, (eds.), *Neuropsychiatry in World War II. Vol. 2: Overseas theaters.* Washington, D.C.: U.S. Government Printing Office, pp. 127–142.
Wiltse, C. M. (1965). *The Medical Department: medical service in the Mediterranean and minor theaters. United States Army in World War II.* Washington, D.C.: U.S. Department of the Army.
Worthington, E. (1977). Post-service adjustment and Vietnam era veterans. *Military Medicine, 142*, 865–866.

3
Soviet Military Psychiatry

RICHARD A. GABRIEL

In order to comprehend Soviet military psychiatry, it is necessary to understand its development against the background of Soviet and Russian military history. Like all things Russian, military psychiatry in its present form has been enormously influenced by the experience of the Russian and Soviet armies on the field of battle. Soviet military history has been marked by the slow learning of past lessons and adopting them gradually in order to develop solutions to modern problems. Accordingly, it is helpful in placing modern Soviet military psychiatry in perspective to be aware of the historical development of Russian military psychiatry from the turn of the century through World War II.

1900–1917

The first army to specifically diagnose mental disease as a consequence of the stresses of modern warfare and to attempt to do something about it was the Russian Army during the Russo-Japanese War of 1905. Prior to this, as with the British in the Boer War and the Americans in the Civil War, soldiers were identified as manifesting behavioral problems that affected their ability to fight. But their problems were most often attributed to factors other than the sheer stress of combat.

During the Russo-Japanese War, physicians in the Russian Army diagnosed and treated approximately two thousand casualties which they directly attributed to battle stress and its resulting psychiatric breakdown. But the number of soldiers complaining of psychiatric symptoms was so large that they overburdened the medical system and were shipped home and turned over to the Russian Red Cross Society for institutionalized care. The number of neuropsychiatric casualties reached such proportions that even home front resources eventually proved to be insufficient. The Russian experience in 1905 provided the first example of "evacuation syndrome" in modern times. When soldiers began to realize that "insane" soldiers were being evacuated, the number of psychiatric casualties increased dramatically as soldiers began to manifest the permitted symptoms in order to gain relief from the stress of battle.

The Russian medical corps seems to have been the first to place psychiatrists relatively close to the battlefront in order to deal with psychiatric breakdown. Most of these psychiatrists, however, came from civilian mental hospitals and had no training in dealing with military psychiatric problems. Psychiatric dispensaries staffed with psychiatrists and other medical personnel were established near the frontlines and had their own transport, usually a specially marked ambulance, to deal with stress casualties as distinct from physical casualties. The dispensary staff often included a neurologist, a feldsher (a physician's assistant), and three sanitors (medics) under the direction of a psychiatrist. Although most Western armies reached this degree of organizational definition by 1917, the principle of "proximity," stationing psychiatric personnel close to the battlefront and treating neuropsychiatric casualties there, was a practical lesson that seems to have been forgotten during the interwar period and did not emerge in practice again until the later days of World War II. However, it was the Russian Army in 1905 that was the first to develop the practice, if not the theoretical underpinning, of a basic premise of military psychiatry: the principle of proximity of treatment.

In the Russo-Japanese War, the Russian Army established a central psychiatric hospital behind the lines in the town of Harbin, Manchuria. This hospital recorded between forty-three and ninety admissions a day for neuropsychiatric casualties. Of these, only a few could be rapidly treated and sent back to the front. Those who remained in the hospital did so for about fifteen days and were subjected to a variety of treatment therapies. If they did not recover, they were evacuated to Moscow by train, a trip that often took forty days because only a single railroad track ran from Harbin to Moscow. Evacuation was accompanied by a surgeon and a small staff of feldshers and, by the end of the war, the Russian medical corps had established a number of special trains exclusively for the use of psychiatric patients. These trains had special isolation compartments, restraint rooms, and barred windows in order to control the patients.

Although the Russians attempted to treat psychiatric casualties at the front; the rates of successful recovery suggest that the treatment was not very successful. Of the 275 officers admitted to the psychiatric hospital in Harbin during the war, only 54 recovered sufficiently to be sent back to the lines and 214 were evacuated to Moscow. Of the 1,072 enlisted soldiers treated in Harbin, only 51 recovered and were returned to their units, whereas 983 were evacuated to the rear. Even in 1905, the Russians began to recognize the problem of secondary gain. They discovered quickly that the further a soldier suffering psychiatric symptoms was evacuated from the front, the less likely he was to recover from his symptoms. Secondary gain was due to a number of factors. In the Russian view, it was due to the perception that stress reactions were often functional for the soldier in that they allowed him to escape the horrors of battle. Once the soldier understood that certain symptoms would allow him to be evacuated out of danger, he began to manifest those symptoms. Moreover, as he was moved further and further away from the battle area, he became less able and willing to reverse those symptoms, so that the further to the rear he went the deeper his symptoms became. The problem of secondary gain became a major problem for Western armies in World War I and II. By the end of World War I, the experience of most Western armies had confirmed the validity of the Russian experience in 1905.

During the Russo-Japanese War, Russian physicians appear to have made significant advances in linking battle stress with certain types of somatic symptoms. An analysis of the diagnoses of hundreds of psychiatric cases during the 1905 war shows that the Russians were already able to diagnose battle stress casualties by categories that are quite modern. Russian psychiatrists recorded cases of hysterical excitement, confused states, fugue states, hysterical blindness, surdomutism, local paralysis, and neurasthenia. Although they understood that these symptoms were related to battle stress, Russian psychiatrists, drawing on their own German medical educations, tended to define the impact of stress in purely physiological terms. Thus, a wide range of battle stress symptoms were attributed to traumatic psychosis of organic origin. In the Russo-Japanese War, 55.6 percent of all battle stress casualties were attributed directly to traumatic damage to the brain or the nervous system.

By the end of the war, and certainly by World War I, the Russian Army probably had the most practical clinical experience with stress casualties insofar as it recognized stress per se as a cause of psychiatric disability. To be sure, by modern Western standards its treatment methods would be regarded as somewhat primitive, but, for their time, they were comparatively advanced. Moreover, the Russo-Japanese War provided physicians in the Russian Army with the first practical opportunity to institutionalize clinical treatment methods for stress casualties deduced directly from the organic and physiological premises of Russian biological psychiatry. Thus, the mold was set for continuing the physiological approach to the treatment of battle stress that would persist until the present in the Soviet Army. Finally, the Russian experience in the Russo-Japanese War established a significant experiential base for institutionalizing the principle of proximity of treatment as a way of dealing with the greater problems of secondary gain.

WORLD WAR I

The Russian Army's experience with battle stress casualties in World War I remains obscure, primarily because events in Russia following the war were so severe and traumatic as to make the collection and publication of information on almost any scientific or medical subject very difficult and, in many cases, impossible. Thus, between 1917 and 1940, the period in which one would have expected that the Russian experience with battle psychiatry in World War I would have finally emerged in print, there is no material available on the subject at all. Neither the international medical journal, *Lancet*, nor the Russian medical journals from 1914 to 1940 contains a single article from any source dealing with the subject of Soviet or Russian military psychiatry or the treatment of neuropsychiatric casualties in World War I.

This does not mean that physicians in the Soviet Army were not thinking about the problems of military psychiatry. In their official histories, which are always to be regarded with some distrust especially in the area of psychiatry, the Soviets note that between 1918 and 1920 three books a year were published on the general subjects of psychology and psychiatry and between 1931 and 1940, seven books a year. Yet, an examination of these works shows that they were all highly theoretical and were more concerned with trying to square Marxist ideology with clinical approaches of military psychiatry than with actual techniques of the discipline. By and large, the works dealt with the psychology of military teaching.

Despite the difficulty in obtaining hard data, we can gain some insight into Soviet psychiatric practice by remembering that much of their medical practice during the war strongly paralleled their own experiences in the Russo-Japanese War. In addition, most Russian psychiatric practice was, basically German psychiatric practice, and many of the techniques that surfaced in World War II were those used by the German Army in World War I. Accordingly, Russian psychiatric practice in World War I probably used such basic German techniques as electric stimulation of paralyzed limbs, water therapy, and rest, and especially folk medicine derivatives and stimulants. They still used these approaches in World War II. Beyond such general statements little more can be said about Russian psychiatric practice in World War I.

WORLD WAR II

Before we can assess the Soviet Army's ability to deal with battle stress casualties in World War II, it is first necessary to establish a baseline against which the data can be analyzed. This task is complicated by the Soviets' traditional secretiveness about their battle performance in the Great Patriotic War and, since 1950, by their effort to rewrite those events to reflect their own version of history. Western military analysts do not know the exact number of men the Soviet Union mobilized for military service in World War II. There is further disagreement on the number of Russian casualties during the war. In his *Encyclopedia of Military History*, T. R. Dupuy states that the Soviets mobilized 25 million men for battle in the war, and, of that number, he suggests that 7.5 million were killed and another 14 million wounded, statistics indicating that almost everyone who served was either killed or wounded (Dupuy, 1970, p. 1198). A second casualty estimate is offered by Lieutenant Colonel Robert Glantz of the Strategic Studies Institute of the U.S. Army War College, Carlisle Barracks, Pennsylvania. Glantz suggests that Dupuy's figures are too high and that the Soviets mobilized about 20 million men, of whom 5 million were killed and between 8 and 9 million were wounded. For purposes of this analysis it seems useful to choose a figure between the two estimates and to use the figure of 22 million as a baseline for determining the number of conscriptions. Of these 22 million, about 20 million were eventually put in uniform.

By contrast, the United States conscripted approximately 20 million men for military service, 14 million of whom passed the initial physical and psychological screening and were eventually pressed into service. Of these 14 million, 260,000 were killed and another 480,000 were wounded on all fronts. In terms of military psychiatry, it is interesting to note that of the 14 million U.S. soldiers about 504,000 suffered psychiatric problems of sufficient magnitude to allow them to obtain a release from military service (Ginzberg, 1959, p. 93).

The Soviets apparently had no formal philosophy or standard of selection except that of obvious physical impairments that would normally exempt the soldier from strenuous exercises as well as combat. Their basic recruitment philosophy was that every Soviet citizen, including women, had to serve in some capacity. There were no nonmedical exemptions from military service, nor were there any psychological or behavioral models used to screen conscripts as was the case in the West. Everyone was expected to serve, and soldiers were assigned where needed and were expected to perform. When they failed to perform, harsh punishments, often death, were imposed. Certainly, the "failure to adapt" to military life, a major reason why conscripts escaped military service in the United States, was not acceptable in the Soviet Army.

In the Soviet Union every citizen fifty-five years old or younger who was physically fit was called to military service. The draft screening procedure centered around a number of local military commissions or commissariats. Each commission was comprised of medical doctors, usually internists and neurologists, who examined conscripts and passed on their general physical health. No psychiatrists served on these boards, and no psychiatric tests were administered. (Even in the modern Soviet Army no psychiatrists serve on the conscript examining boards.)

Whatever psychiatric screening was done was on an ad hoc basis and was accomplished by neurologists whose physiological orientation permitted them to detect any organic causes that might be responsible for behavioral problems. Only those who suffered from imbecillia or were obviously psychotic were allowed to escape military service for other than clear physical disabilities. The number of conscripts who were deferred from military service on purely psychiatric grounds was very small indeed. Problems of neurosis were not regarded as serious enough to merit exemption and, to date are not viewed as serious enough to defer a Soviet conscript. Rejections for psychiatric reasons were not a major cause of military manpower loss to the Soviets in World War II.

It is somewhat easier to obtain data on the number of rejections for psychiatric reasons which the Soviets allowed in World War II. To be sure, the data are not definitive, having been obtained by interviewing a number of medical doctors and neurologists who served on draft medical commissions during the war; some served as battle surgeons later on. According to these sources, of the 22 million men who were conscripted, only a small number, perhaps no more than 50,000 to 75,000, were exempted from military service for purely psychiatric problems. This constitutes a rejection rate of less than 0.25 percent. Even at the extreme, the figure would not exceed 1 percent of the total pool examined. By comparison, the United States examined some 18 million men and rejected 5,250,000, or about 29 percent of the total pool for "mental, moral, and physical" reasons. The United States found 71 percent of its conscript pool fit for military duty, or approximately 12,750,000 men. It rejected 970,000 for neuropsychiatric disorders and other emotional problems. Thus, psychiatric reasons accounted for 18.5 percent of those rejected for military service. As a percentage of the total conscript pool, 5.4 percent of those initially screened for military service were rejected for psychiatric disorders (Ginzberg, 1959, p. 35). This rejection rate was twenty times greater than that in the Soviet Army.

In attempting to determine the Soviets' success in reducing the loss of soldiers in battle units as a consequence of neuropsychiatric breakdown, we must remember that the degree to which military units will generate neuropsychiatric casualties in the first place depends on a number of factors, not all of which are directly quantifiable (unit cohesion, quality of leadership, replacement system, and so on). Yet, three major factors that are directly related to the rates at which units will generate psychiatric casualties are the type of battle a unit must fight, its intensity, and its duration. In this regard the Soviets fought almost five long years of war, much of it under conditions of disarray and near collapse. Moreover, the intensity of combat, the size of the battles, and their duration were, on balance, much greater than those experienced by American and British troops, with the possible exception of the Normandy invasion and the battle for Normandy in July 1944. The Soviet Army suffered more physical casualties than any other combatant—perhaps as many as 8 million dead and another 15 million wounded. On this basis alone, Soviet military units could be expected to have generated very high numbers of neuropsychiatric casualties.

The number of psychiatric casualties among Soviet soldiers can also be related to the manner in which they conducted battle. A study done by Lieutenant Colonel Robert Glantz of the Strategic Studies Institute at the U.S. Army War College based on an analysis of hundreds of Soviet combat unit histories and diaries concludes that Soviet divisions typically went into battle at only 70 percent strength in manpower and equipment. Another quite common practice was to fight these units down to 25 percent and 30 percent strength before stopping the attack. Even then Soviet units were seldom pulled out of the line. Instead, they would throw another division into the breach, joining the remaining elements of the bloodied unit to the new one and then continuing the attack. These practices suggest that the tempo of war was very intense for Soviet units and that Soviet battle doctrine itself probably increased what was an already high level of combat deaths, wounds, and stress casualties.

Because the rate of psychiatric casualties generated by units is related to the intensity, duration, and type of battle, and because it tends to vary directly with the number of killed and wounded suffered by a unit, Soviet units in World War II may well have suffered high rates of neuropsychiatric casualties. It is, of course, impossible to determine the exact rate, for no data are available. As we will see, we may determine the number of soldiers lost to units as a result of such casualties. The rates of initial psychiatric breakdown in Soviet units were likely at least as high as in the American Army and, in all probability, much higher.

The challenge of military psychiatry is not so much how to prevent psychiatric breakdown among men engaged in battle but to learn the mechanisms that produce psychiatric breakdown in battle. Military psychiatry's practical task is to treat as many cases as quickly as possible and to return them to their units in order to preserve the army's manpower strength. The most significant overall test of military psychiatry, the cultural values of the various combatants aside, is the degree to which it can stop or reduce manpower loss to fighting units. By this standard, Soviet military psychiatry seems to have done very well during World War II.

In World War II the Soviet Army mobilized approximately 22 million men, of whom 5 million were killed and another 9 million wounded. This means that at least 14 million men saw direct combat, although the figure is realistically higher. Based on more than a score of interviews with Soviet combat doctors, including psychiatrists and neurologists, it is possible to estimate the number of Soviet soldiers who were diagnosed as suffering from psychiatric problems serious enough to warrant evacuation from their units. The Red Army's loss rate for neuropsychiatric reasons was under ten per thousand and probably closer to six per thousand. This is about the same rate suffered by the American Army in World War I. If we use this figure as a baseline, during World War II the Soviet Army suffered between 96,000 and 100,000 psychiatric casualties that were eventually classed as manpower losses.

The American Army alone (not counting army air crews, naval, or Marine casualties) suffered a total of 504,000 separations from military service as a result of psychiatric problems. Of these, 333,000 were true neuropsychiatric cases of psychosis and psychoneurosis. The difference between the two figures, 171,000, is attributable to separations from service resulting from "behavioral problems" and the "failure to adapt" to military life (Ginzberg, 1959, p. 61). Only 42 percent of the total number of separations for psychiatric reasons in the American forces in World War II occurred among men who actually faced the enemy. Amazingly, 58 percent of the psychiatric separations occurred in the zone of interior, that is, in the United States before these men were ever sent overseas or into battle! (See Ginzberg, 1959, p. 100).

Of the 333,000 separations resulting from psychosis and psychoneurosis that occurred in combat zones, among those soldiers who saw ground combat duty in Europe alone the rate of psychiatric casualty loss was thirty-eight per thousand. This means that the ground combat army suffered approximately 12,616 neuropsychiatric casualties that were severe enough to be removed from the combat pool for the duration of the war. This figure does not include the thousands who broke down in battle, were treated, and eventually returned to their units. During World War II approximately 40 percent of the soldiers who suffered psychiatric breakdown were successfully returned to their units. If one examines the ratio of psychiatric casualties to the number of dead and wounded, American ground forces suffered 234,874 dead and 568,861 men wounded. Thus, the ratio of psychiatric casualties to wounded was 1 to 19, whereas the ratio of psychiatric casualties to killed in action was 1 to 43.

These figures suggest that, whereas the Soviet Army may have suffered higher initial rates of psychiatric casualties (they suffered a higher absolute number of such casualties) than did the American Army, once these casualties occurred, the Soviet medical system was able to minimize the rate of manpower loss to fighting units by treating psychiatric patients and keeping them on the frontlines. The overall rates of return show that the loss rate owing to psychiatric casualties in the American Army was four to six times higher than that in the Soviet Army. Moreover, the ratio of psychiatric casualties to dead was 2.5 times higher than that in the Soviet Army, whereas the rate of psychiatric casualties to wounded was twice as high.

What policies, doctrines, and practices enabled the Soviet Army to sustain its manpower strength during World War II by keeping psychiatric casualty losses to a minimum? One factor was the manner in which the Soviets perceived the causes of battle-shock and were prepared to deal with it.

In the Soviet view, soldiers who manifested battle-shock symptoms were making a functional adjustment to their environment. That is, soldiers who wished to escape the horrors of the battlefield were essentially normal, sane people who were prepared to go to great lengths to escape their environment. The values of the Soviet military subculture defined what types of behavior it would permit. These values, in turn, framed a set of expectations for both the controllers of the military subsystem and its participants. As one might expect of a totalitarian and ideologically motivated military system, the Soviet view of battle-shock was extremely harsh.

In the Soviet lexicon, "shock" is equivalent to the Russian term "udar," the same term used to describe a heart attack, epileptic stroke, or even an electrical shock. There is no clinical term for "battle-shock."

SOVIET MILITARY PSYCHIATRY

The Soviets use the term "reaction" for psychological symptoms with no accompanying physical cause. They regard such "reactions" as problems of small psychiatry. The Russian term for shock delineates a condition that is physiologically caused, has physiological symptoms, and is subject to physiological cure. The Soviet view does not admit of a condition of psychiatric breakdown that is induced as a consequence of purely emotional and psychological factors for which there is no accompanying physiological cause. Even in the diagnosis of schizophrenia and severe psychosis, Soviet biological psychiatry places the eventual cause of such diseases in some organic disruption of the brain. In World War II the Soviets did not regard emotional trauma per se as a legitimate excuse for permitting the soldier relief from battle. The only legitimate excuse allowed the soldier suffering from stress was a symptomology that had a clearly discernible physiological cause resulting from injury.

The Soviets maintain that combat shock is organically caused and, therefore, may be corrected by treating the patient's damaged or disrupted physiology. Those purely emotional or psychic causes which in the United States would be regarded as expected consequences of battlefield stress are regarded by Soviet psychiatrists as shortcomings in the soldier's character, motivation, or training. The fact that a soldier may be too frightened to move, suffer tremors, have difficulty processing information, be reluctant to fire his weapon, or any number of other symptoms, which in the American Army would be regarded as significant indicators of battle stress, are, in the Soviet Army, not taken seriously. They view conditions such as fear, anxiety, and tremors as normal conditions that develop on the battlefield, and they place the responsibility for dealing with them and continuing to function squarely on the soldier.

The Soviets regard a soldier who suffers abnormally high levels of anxiety, fear, or panic as an individual who either has a defect in his character or is suffering from problems of improper motivation, morale, and training. Responsibility for failures of morale and motivation is placed not only on the soldier, but also on the unit commander and most particularly on the political officer. The Soviets refuse to address what, in the United States, would be regarded as normal symptoms of battle stress as a medical problem.

Accordingly, in World War II, the Soviets refused to admit that a whole range of psychiatric casualites were in fact psychiatric casualties at all. Instead of treating these casualties in the medical and evacuation chain, they were turned over to unit commanders and political officers to be dealt with on a motivational basis. By refusing to recognize the validity of neuropsychiatric symptoms, the Soviets were able to prevent the evacuation of large numbers of soldiers who manifested these symptoms and to hold them in the battlezone much longer. Only physically based symptoms or cases of obvious psychosis were taken seriously as medical problems.

In World War II, Soviet psychiatrists distinguished between what they called "big psychiatry" and "small psychiatry" in their attempt to diagnose psychiatric problems. Problems of big psychiatry referred to illnesses associated with organic disorders or disruptions of the brain and tended largely to focus on schizophrenia and the other major psychoses. Big psychiatry focused on those behavioral manifestations that could be traced to organic injuries caused largely by some sort of commotion, concussion, or contusion leading to organic brain damage to include neurologic injuries to the spinal cord. Almost all other symptoms shown by combat soldiers—fear, anxiety, tremors, inability to sleep, partial paralysis, and a range of other symptoms—were regarded as problems of small psychiatry normally diagnosed in a range of temporary to permanent neurosis. Problems of small psychiatry were dealt with not by psychiatrists but by unit commanders, political officers, and, in more severe cases, neurologists.

Each battalion had a political officer whose task was to ensure the motivation, morale, and fighting spirit of his unit. At battalion level, the political officer often had a small staff that went into the companies and carried out similar tasks. When soldiers failed to demonstrate the proper motivation and morale, failed to perform correctly, or began to manifest symptoms normally associated with combat stress, Soviet units had someone in place who dealt immediately with the problem. The presence of the political officer within the unit, accompanied by a comparatively harsh doctrine that strictly defined and limited the symptoms that would qualify as a legitimate reason to evacuate a soldier from the front, led the Soviets to apply two of the basic principles of combat psychiatry, namely, expectancy and proximity of treatment. These two principles applied most directly to the range of problems associated with small psychiatry. The result was a low rate of manpower loss to combat units as a consequence of psychiatric problems.

It produced a much lower rate of manpower loss for these reasons than was incurred by the U.S. Army.

Although harsh by U.S. standards, the Soviet system worked very well. In extreme cases threats of execution were used and sometimes carried out. Soviet battlefield discipline in World War II was extremely strict, and the execution of a soldier who failed to perform was regarded as merely company punishment which required no trial or hearing. And there were enough battlefield executions of soldiers who would not perform adequately to give credence to the threat. If one was not shot, then a soldier would be sent to a penal battalion where he would endure a much harsher life with a greater chance of being killed than even at the frontline. Assignments to penal battalions meant certain combat under the most difficult and often suicidal conditions.

Soviet military psychiatry employed a strict definition of the "ticket out," the set of symptoms required before a soldier was allowed to be evacuated from the frontlines. The Soviet ticket out was defined in nonpsychic, almost neurological terms requiring some physical cause—commotion, contusion, concussion, or other traumatic injury to the brain or spinal cord—that could be blamed for the soldier's behavioral problem. Not only did the Soviets require that the cause of the problem be organically based, but most often the diagnostic screen also required that the behavioral symptomology be accompanied by a physiological effect such as paralysis, bleeding from the ears or nose, hysteria, or surdomutism. Soldiers with no physiological elements of diagnosis were regarded as shirkers and cowards and were to be dealt with as such.

Because it was assumed that a soldier's problems were caused by organic damage accompanied by distinct physical symptoms that could be traced to this damage, Soviet medical personnel assumed that both symptoms and causes could be treated much more readily than was generally the case in the United States. The Soviets assumed from the beginning—no doubt drawing on their experience in the Russo-Japanese War and World War I—that the organic causes of psychiatric problems required rapid treatment close to the battlefront. Thus, Soviet combat psychiatry in World War II was based not only on the principles of proximity and expectancy, but also on the third principle of military psychiatry, immediacy of treatment. Because the causes of psychiatric debilitation were seen to be traceable to organic injury. Soviet treatment tended to stress physical methodologies. As a consequence, psychiatrists could avoid dealing with the soldier's psyche and other emotional problems and could deal directly with the soldier's body and brain. This made the provision of treatment close to the front comparatively easy, more rapid, and, in fact, seems to have increased the probability of recovery.

The medical system for dealing with psychiatric casualties set a high and diagnostically precise price for excusing a soldier from battle. Many of the reasons allowed in Western armies were regarded as a soldier's normal reactions in battle and were *ab initio* defined as insufficient to relieve the soldier from the fighting. Soldiers suffering from severe stress symptoms might be granted a short period of rest at the battalion or regimental aid station. But, in general, their symptoms were not regarded as sufficient cause to evacuate them further to the rear.

The Soviet medical evacuation system in World War II was extremely primitive, when it existed at all, and did not operate consistently. The initial suspicion with which psychiatric symptoms were met, coupled with few mechanisms for diagnosing psychiatric casualties with no accompanying physical damage, when added to a medical evacuation system that was barely functional, meant that, fewer psychiatric cases got into the evacuation train to begin with. The Soviet medical evacuation system was not willing to evacuate anyone without serious physical injury, and so most psychiatric casualties were retained for longer periods within the battlezone where they were treated by unit commanders, political officers, sanitors, feldshers, and regimental surgeons.

The Soviet approach to neuropsychiatric casualties during the war was reflected in the structure of medical care and treatment. A basic fact that emerges from an analysis of the Soviet medical structure is the lack of formal psychiatric training among medical personnel below regimental level. Indeed, there were no psychiatrists or psychiatric treatment staff at division level, a condition that was common in Western armies during World War II and that had existed in some armies since World War I.

At the army and front levels, however, there were special hospitals and staff for dealing with psychiatric patients. At the front-level hospital, located about 100 miles to the rear of the fighting, often a complete psychiatric hospital and a staff of six to eight psychiatrists and neurologists were attached to the usual surgical hospital. Psychiatric patients were treated by psychiatrists and neurologists, although, once again, the bulk of the treatment seems to have been directed by neurologists focusing on the organic cause of the behavioral problem. The front-level hospital had facilities for about 100 psychiatric patients.

Closer to the fighting was the army-level hospital located between 50 and 75 miles from the battle. This facility had a small psychiatric ward capable of accommodating forty patients. Yet, only some of these beds were actually set aside for psychiatric patients. The psychiatric staff of the army-level hospital consisted of two to three doctors. Sometimes army-level hospitals had no psychiatrists at all but relied on neurologists to treat patients. Usually, however, at least one psychiatrist was in residence. This tendency to mix psychiatrists and neurologists has a long history in Soviet psychiatric practice and is based on the assumption that behavioral aberrations are due essentially to organic disruptions of the brain and nervous system.

At division level there were no provisions at all for psychiatrists or psychiatric staffs. The division had a basic medical battalion that provided normal casualty treatment support to the division. Below division were doctors located at the regimental aid station which supplemented the division aid station. Many of the doctors at regimental level were neurologists, but most of them were battle surgeons ranging from trained surgeons to general practitioners. Below regiment was the battalion aid station staffed by a feldsher and a few medics and, lower still, at company level, was only the normal complement of company medics. Thus, at division or below, the Soviet Army made no provisions for treating psychiatric casualties. As one moved further toward the front, one found fewer and fewer medical personnel of any sort. Moreover, in the training of Soviet medical personnel below division no effort was made to incorporate any knowledge of combat psychiatry.

Being untrained in psychiatric diagnosis, lower level medical personnel tended to reinforce the system's predominant tendency to regard certain kinds of behavior as either normal consequences of fear, defects in character, or in other ways that the system itself had defined them. Rather than shunting such patients into the medical evacuation chain, they were kept in the command and administrative chain and were diverted, as the system was designed to do, to commissars and unit commanders to be dealt with accordingly.

The Soviet military reinforced this practice by regarding high rates of psychiatric casualties within a unit as the result of a breakdown of command and leadership, placing the responsibility directly on the unit commander. Every battalion and regiment had a political officer who was directly responsible for the morale, motivation, and ideological fighting strength of his unit. High levels of psychiatric casualties were seen as the political officer's failure to do his job. Paradoxically, although the Soviet system did not formally assign psychiatrists and other clinically trained personnel to lower unit levels to aid in the diagnosis and treatment of psychiatric casualties, in practice the system worked as well as if they did. By charging both the unit commander and the political officer with maintaining the fighting spirit of his unit and then holding them rigorously responsible for any failures in this spirit (especially psychiatric casualties), the commander and commissar acquired a strong personal interest in keeping the rates of evacuation for psychiatric reasons to a minimum. They were forced to deal with such problems quickly and on the spot or face the prospect of serious consequences themselves.

Soviet commanders and medical personnel understood, however, that some categories of psychiatric illness were so severe that they had to be recognized for what they were. In instances of genuine psychosis, soldiers were evacuated rapidly. In these cases the task of the feldshers, medics, and battalion surgeons was to diagnose the truly psychotic from those who were suffering from only "normal" combat reactions or problems of small psychiatry. Individuals suffering from normal combat reactions were treated as close to their fighting units as possible. At each stage of the evacuation, depending on how serious the problem was, psychiatric patients were given lower priority than physical casualties, and they were often shunted aside at battalion, regimental, or division aid stations where they were allowed to rest until they could be examined more thoroughly. Usually, after a few days' rest even soldiers with the most severe nonpsychotic combat reactions were returned to the fighting. Truly psychotic individuals, on the other hand, were immediately removed from their fighting units and isolated until evacuation could be accomplished. As they moved further to the rear, at each stage they were isolated until they could be treated. By limiting evacuation to those psychiatric cases with extreme and obvious symptoms, the Soviets were able to keep the number of soldiers lost as psychiatric casualties to a minimum. During World War I the

U.S. Army used a similarly conservative definition for evacuating psychiatric casualties and much the same evacuation procedure. The rates of manpower loss to psychiatric causes for the U.S. Army in World War I and for the Soviet Army in World War II were about the same—approximately six to nine per thousand.

The Soviets were able to reduce the level of battle-shock casualties by narrowing the diagnostic definition of a neuropsychiatric casualty. Soviet psychiatrists drew on their previous experience in physiology and neurology and even more so on the Germanic psychiatric tradition of locating behavioral problems in the physiological disruption of the brain. Not surprisingly, the treatment of battle-shock was a continuation of the biological approach to psychiatry that had been evident in Russia since at least 1860. On the battlefield psychiatrists sustained the belief that behavioral aberration had a physical cause, usually "brain shock" or, more clinically, traumatic encephalopathy. This implied some sort of brain damage which interfered with proper function varying in duration. The basic diagnostic assumption was that soldiers suffering from behavioral problems, psychosis, and even neuroses of some type were suffering from organic brain damage.

Soviet psychiatrists focused on what they called concussion, commotion, and contusion of the brain, which was usually associated with loss of consciousness, as a major cause of overt behavioral symptoms. This focus accurately reflects the terminology which the French used in World War I to explain psychiatric reactions to battle stress. In more precise terms, Soviet psychiatrists, being first and foremost medical doctors educated in the Germanic tradition of biological psychiatry, attributed behavioral aberrations to bruising of the brain, microbleeding in the interior of the brain, the presence of brain lesions, edema, and microscopic scars caused by trauma or disease. The approach was to attempt to link the soldier's overt behavioral symptoms—paralysis, mutism, blindness, and so on—to the damage that may have been done to certain areas of the brain.

According to 44 personal interviews conducted with Soviet doctors who served in World War II, Soviet soldiers suffered a very high rate of conversion reactions. This situation would not be unexpected, for soldiers respond to the expectations and cultural norms of the military subculture to which they belong. They respond to precisely those symptoms which the system defines as acceptable for escaping stress. With Soviet psychiatrists having defined the "ticket out" of battle as being related to brain damage causing overt physiological manifestations, soldiers began to convert their fears and anxieties into precisely these manifestations.

Once the troops discovered that certain symptomologies associated with traumatic encephalopathy were "successful" in permitting a soldier to escape his stressful environment, they began to develop these symptomologies as a truly functional way of dealing with stress. This phenomenon is a familiar one among other armies with different sets of acceptable symptoms. Soviet psychiatry regarded such adjustments as patently explainable because they believed any adjustment to stress not caused by a genuine organic disruption was functional insofar as it served to remove the "organism" from a stressful environment. Consequently, such conversion reactions as hysteria, deafness and dumbness, surdomutism, partial paralysis, and fugue states,—all familiar to Western combat psychiatrists—were common.

Soviet neurologists point out that the rate of conversion reactions became so high in the Soviet Army that doctors and other field medical personnel had to develop shorthand tests to determine which conversion reactions were genuine, which symptoms were tied to organic damage, and which were shallow enough to qualify as faking. Most of these tests were simple and seemed to have worked quite well. Many were drawn from similar treatments used by the German Army and other Western armies in World War I. No doubt the Russian Army also used a number of them in World War I.

One of the most commonly used techniques was the Kaufmann method invented by French psychiatrists and used by the German Army in World War I. The test had actually been developed before World War I in civilian clinical applications and had been taught at Russian medical schools before the war. It was a specific treatment for dealing with patients suffering from surdomutism. The object of the treatment was to force the patient to speak as a way of breaking the syndrome. Electrodes were placed on the patient's throat, and moderately intense and painful electrical current was administered. The patient was told that the point of the treatment was to reestablish the damaged pathways from his throat to his brain. In truth, Soviet psychiatrists probably did not believe this. What they were trying to do was to shock the brain, as in electro-convulsive therapy (which was also used in other cases) into acting normally again. From the patient's perspective, it often seemed that the choice came down to sustaining his symptoms by enduring a considerable amount of pain or abandoning his symptoms as a way of ridding himself of the pain. This method was also used to treat patients suffering from partial paralysis, a common occurrence widely seen in Western armies in World War I. The paralysis often took the form of contractive paralysis of the arm needed to operate the bolt of the soldier's weapon. Electric stimulation was administered directly to the affected limb.

Another method for dealing with conversion reactions was to place a rubberized mask over the patient's face and to gradually induce a feeling of suffocation. This technique was used to treat soldiers suffering from fugue states, inability to speak, and paralysis. Again the object was to force the patient to choose between sustaining his symptoms under great discomfort and relinquishing his symptoms by making some physical effort or crying out to remove the mask. The premise behind the test was that only those whose conditions were traceable to organic injury would be able to tolerate suffocation until they lost consciousness. A variation of the technique was to wrap a rag around the patient's face and pour water on it to simulate the feeling of drowning in the hope that he would respond. Still another test was to poke the soldier's paralyzed limbs with needles in order to produce enough pain to get him to respond with movement. Not uncommonly, soldiers in fugue states or deep conversion states were able to sustain the pain and discomfort administered. Soldiers in fugue states were often tested by the simple device of making a sudden loud noise and watching for physiological reactions which would prove that the state was not induced by true organic damage. These few tests were used extensively by medical personnel at all levels of the medical treatment system, but seem to have been used most commonly by doctors at the army and division levels as a way of determining whether the soldier's condition was due to organic damage or brain disruption. Soviet psychiatrists and doctors report that in a large number of cases, especially after the soldier had a few days of rest away from the fighting, these treatments met with success.

Only the most severe combat reactions or truly psychotic patients were evacuated out of combat. But even when faced with genuine psychiatric problems, the tendency was not to evacuate a patient beyond division if it could be avoided. The doctors and commanders feared that once a patient was evacuated for purely psychiatric reasons, other soldiers would be encouraged to develop similar symptoms. Thus, every effort was made to find some assignment for the soldier so that he could continue to serve. Even rest was normally accomplished within the general zone of fighting.

The key to the effectiveness of the Soviet system of dealing with battle reactions was effective screening at the lower levels and convincing the soldier in advance that certain types of psychiatric problems would not be permitted. When a soldier began to manifest psychiatric symptoms, he would be screened immediately by a medic or by his unit commander. If the problem could not be handled here, the soldier was sent to the battalion or company aid station, where a decision was made whether to send him to his political officer or back to his unit commander because his problem usually was not serious enough. If the issue was in doubt, the soldier would be allowed to rest for a short time, about twenty-four hours, at the battalion aid station. If symptoms persisted, he was sent to regiment for examination where he would be given a number of "curative psychiatric tests" to see if his symptoms could be abated. If there was no physiological damage to the brain or spinal cord, the soldier might be allowed to remain at regiment for a few days of rest where he was assigned to a minor job. Above regiment, only the most severe psychiatric cases were evacuated.

As in any army, when heavy combat occurred the system of casualty treatment and evacuation broke down. Medical support in the Soviet Army in World War II was primitive to begin with, and, when large numbers of casualties occurred, the system's ability to deal with them declined rapidly. Under these conditions, the Soviet Army reacted differently in its treatment of psychiatric casualties than did most Western armies. In the West, for example, when heavy casualties overwhelmed the medical system, soldiers manifesting symptoms of psychiatric breakdown were often placed in the medical chain and evacuated to the rear rather than being detained and treated at the front. This practice further taxed the entire evacuation and treatment system. The Soviets reacted differently. When casualties became heavy, those suffering from psychiatric problems were treated even more harshly. In general, if a soldier could walk and had no obvious physical wound, he was immediately turned back to the fighting. In addition, special military police units conducted regular patrols through the medical aid stations, gathering up stragglers or soldiers who were not wounded and forcing them back into the line. As a consequence, when physical casualties increased, the number of psychiatric evacuations actually decreased—exactly the opposite of what happened in most Western armies.

During World War II the only soldiers who received serious treatment from psychiatrists where those who were evacuated back to army-level hospitals. The treatments administered at army- and front-level hospitals were essentially the same as those used by the French and Germans in World War I. The American and British armies had used a number of treatments in that war as well. A psychiatric casualty sent to an army-level hospital had a normal stay of two weeks for "mild" cases, three weeks for moderate cases, and up to six weeks for the most severe cases. Those who recovered in this time were sent back to the front. For the most part, the Soviets did not make great efforts to return recovered soldiers to their units. The Soviets realized that their practice of fighting units down to the nub would result in very high casualties to combat units, and, as such, they probably did not see much value in attempting to return soldiers to units which, in many cases, had been decimated or destroyed while the patient was recovering in the hospital. In some instances, Soviet front commanders actually prohibited the practice of sending men back to their units, although a number of Soviet soldiers report instances of recovered soldiers fleeing replacement depots in attempts to find comrades in their old units. The Soviets did not use a unit replacement system during the war, as did the Germans and British, but instead adopted an individual replacement system built around replacement depots that strongly resembled the system used by the United States.

Interviews with Soviet neurologists, psychiatrists, and surgeons who worked at army-level hospitals suggest that the Soviets were able to return well over 80 percent of the cases held in psychiatric wards, a figure twice as high as the 40 percent returned by the American Army. Furthermore, the 80 percent who were returned did so within six to eight weeks of being evacuated, a comparatively short time to return severe cases of psychiatric debilitation. In institutionalizing mechanisms to locate, examine, and then return recovered neuropsychiatric casualties to the line, the Soviet Army was practicing a basic principle of military psychiatry—the principle of expectancy. The Soviet soldier expected that no matter what else happened, unless he was so severely wounded that he could no longer function at all, he would be returned to battle.

Diagnostically, the Soviets reported a number of severe conversion reactions among Western armies in World War I, including severe hysteria, surdomutism, paralysis, blindness, and others. They also encountered severe depression psychosis sometimes accompanied by memory loss, schizophasia, severe tremors and convulsions, and inability to control body functions. Because the Soviet "ticket out" was defined in physiological terms, most of the symptomology emerged in these terms. They also found that the highest rates of psychiatric casualties were found among infantrymen, whereas soldiers in the armored corps comprised the second largest category. Soviet psychiatrists did not find this unusual, for infantrymen are often subjected to artillery bombardments that cause contusions and concussions. Armor troops often were banged around inside their machines and lost consciousness. At army-level hospitals soldiers who did not recover after six weeks were sent rearward to the front-level hospitals where the same time schedule for recovery used at the army-level hospital obtained. Generally, very few psychiatric casualties recovered at front-level, and most were placed in the civilian public health system (such as it was!) where they were normally discharged from the military.

Treatment of neuropsychiatric casualties at army- and front-level hospitals involved the use of drugs. Perhaps the term "drugs" is an inadequate term if one means relatively sophisticated chemical agents that can be used to treat specific brain disorders with some precision. More correctly, Soviet psychiatrists relied on a range of plant and animal derivatives that were in the category of folk medicines. Authentic drugs such as chloryl hydrate and barbiturates were also used, but no army had sophisticated drugs for use in the treatment of psychiatric problems.

With this caveat, one can point to a range of folk medicines, usually plant and animal derivatives, that Soviet psychiatrists found helpful in dealing with battle-shock cases. Inasmuch as Soviet psychiatric doctrine assumed a physiological cause for psychiatric disruption, the use of chemical compounds to treat the damage to the brain made good sense. A common treatment, also found in the West, required the administration of chloryl hydrate to induce long periods of sleep as part of general rest therapy. Early in the war Soviet psychiatrists, as did many psychiatrists in other armies, learned that even the most severe manifestations of combat shock, including reactive psychosis, would often respond well to concentrated sleep. To induce sleep, chloryl hydrate drops were frequently used, and the results were often dramatic and rapid.

Another treatment involved the use of what Soviet physicians called "brom" or bromide, which was also being used in the United States at the same time. It took the form of either natrium bromide or sodium bromide administered intravenously. It calmed the patient down, putting him into a shallow sedative state. It was also widely used to build up body fluids and to treat brain concussions, contusions, and seizures. Bromide use was discontinued in the United States after World War II, when it was found that it sometimes caused brain damage.

Other herbal medicine compounds used by Soviet psychiatrists were valeriana or valadium, ginseng, powdered reindeer horn, goldroot, and mandarin root, all of which were sedatives or stimulants. The Soviets made extensive use of aloe which they used in liquid form and administered subcutaneously. In the United States, aloe has recently been used in suntan lotion and for the treatment of insect bites and minor burns. The Soviets found it useful in treating a range of traumatic brain injuries and in preventing the formation of scar tissue in the brain after concussions and contusions. Doctors report that an excellent treatment for preventing and treating small brain lesions was a compound called fibs. This natural compound was made from a special mud, refined to a liquid and injected subcutaneously.

Two other treatments used by Soviet psychiatrists were magnesium and calcium chloride administered intravenously. Magnesium IVs were used as a sedative that was also useful in combating brain edema. It controlled the dosage for long periods of time, inducing a sedative effect on the patient without excessive disruption of the body's chemistry. Calcium chloride, a general stimulant, was administered in IV form and was used to gradually raise the patient's excitation level without inducing shock. This treatment was used extensively in dealing with stupor, fugue states, neurasthenia, or cases in which patients could not be brought back to full consciousness. Two treatments used extensively in the United States, narcohypnosis and abreaction, were used only rarely in the Soviet military. Soviet psychiatrists reported these techniques as usually taking too long to work, when they worked at all.

Soviet military psychiatry remained much the same as it had during the war until 1967 when it received renewed emphasis from the military interested in matching Western research and advances. Immediately after the war, Soviet military medical personnel conducted a thorough review of their medical experiences and published it in a multivolume work. One complete volume was prepared on the subject of military psychiatry. By 1967 Soviet military psychiatrists apparently realized that some of the problems of small psychiatry probably needed more study, especially in light of the Soviet military's desire to develop a method of preventing combat shock in the new nuclear battlefield. After the war, several psychiatrists and, after 1967, some psychologists, received grants from the military to study the problems of small psychiatry as they relate to battle stress.

Most of the work being done in the area of preventing and treating battle-shock in a nuclear environment has been restricted to research settings. The few existing applications have been directed at pilots, submariners, astronauts, and other highly skilled technicians in an effort to control fear and anxiety and prevent degradation of performance. With regard to military psychiatry in the ground combat forces, the experiences of World War II have conveyed the message to the military medical establishment that their mechanisms of diagnosis and treatment worked adequately. They have, of course, tried to keep abreast of more modern treatment methods, especially the revolution in psychopharmacology which began in France in the 1950s, and have attempted to incorporate some of these developments in their own treatment methodologies.

The Soviets regard their experience with military psychiatry in World War II as superior to the Western experience in dealing with the same problem. They continue to believe that a strict definition of an acceptable level of traumatic stress can in itself prevent large numbers of psychiatric casualties. This doctrine is still strongly enforced by unit commanders, political officers, and a medical establishment that refuses to recognize psychiatric debilitation that is not clearly tied to physical injury. The Soviet system of treating psychiatric casualties is based on the same practical principles of proximity, immediacy, and expectancy that underpin Western military psychiatry.

MODERN SOVIET MILITARY PSYCHIATRY

Among the more common tasks performed by military psychiatrists in Western armies is screening conscripts for military service. It will be recalled that during World War II the Soviets examined approximately 22 million conscripts for military service. Fewer than 100,000 (and perhaps fewer than 75,000) were rejected for purely psychiatric reasons. No exemptions or releases were granted for "unsuitability" or "failure to adapt," as was commonly the case in the American Army. Conscripts were given standard military physical examinations which focused on finding any debilitating diseases of the heart, lungs, circulatory system, nutritional problems, and other basic categories of physical weakness. Less than 1 percent of all Soviet conscripts were rejected for military service for these reasons. In a practical sense, the Soviet Army impressed almost every conscript it examined.

With regard to draft screening today, the Soviet military psychiatrist has a much smaller role than his Western counterpart and, in many cases, practically none. In dealing with conscripts who might manifest psychiatric problems, a Soviet draft board (draft commissariat) is provided with a list of all patients undergoing psychiatric care within the relevant military district. The civilian public health system is structurally parallel to the military district and commissariat system used for conscription. If the civilian health clinic diagnoses a conscript as having a serious problem or a history of psychiatric illness, the conscript usually is not even called by the military for an examination. Those with marginal or recent histories of mental disturbances are examined by the usual team of military doctors comprised of internists and neurologists. Sometimes a psychiatrist takes extra time to determine if a conscript is faking. Soldiers without any mental history are given perfunctory neurological examinations that are rather similar to those given to U.S. conscripts. No battery of psychiatric tests is administered to conscripts by psychiatrists, or does there appear to be any systematic use of psychiatric questionnaires.

Every civilian health district within the Soviet Union has a neuropsychiatric dispensary that keeps records on all patients within the district with psychotic or severe neurotic mental health problems. The clinics were established in the mid-1920s. In the mid-1970s the Ministry of Mental Health and the Institute of Forensic Psychiatry established a project to computerize all information on every patient in the country who had been treated within the public health system, with special emphasis on psychiatric conditions. A centralized computer file is now being maintained on all psychiatric patients. The basic diagnostic categories used are those used by ICD-9, the commonly recognized, international diagnostic manual widely used in the West. Furthermore, an effort is being made to enforce these diagnostic categories on psychiatric practitioners within the district and dispensary hospitals as a way of imposing some unification on the diagnostic criteria used by the civilian and military authorities in dealing with psychiatric cases. The goal is to develop a common diagnostic terminology that will be functional for both sets of authorities.

In 1980 the Institute of Forensic Psychiatry conducted a study of the military's psychiatric screening procedures as well as the basic psychiatric applications of the national public health system. They discovered two interesting facts. First, on a nationwide basis, the level of diagnosed cases of schizophrenia in each mental health district tended to vary directly with the number of psychiatrists who were present within each mental health district. The greater the number of psychiatrists present in each district, the greater the number of diagnosed cases of schizophrenia. Second, in their study of draft rejections for psychiatric reasons the Institute found that the highest rates of draft rejections for psychiatric reasons were in the Baltic republics of Latvia, Estonia, and Lithuania. The highest rate was in Lithuania where the rejection rate was eight times higher than for any other Soviet republic. The most common diagnostic reason for these rejections was oligophrenia which, in the Soviet lexicon, may be generally translated as mental retardation or "dull-wittedness." (In World War I, one of the most common causes of rejection in the American Army was for a similar condition then defined as "imbecillia.")

Soviet military authorities assume that a sizable number of people will attempt to fake mental or physical problems as a way of escaping military service. In order to deal with the inventiveness of conscripts, Soviet doctors often segregate soldiers who manifest specific symptoms that are apparently false or self-induced. Soviet doctors typically treat the symptoms in such a way as to make the complaints worse. For example, soldiers who complained of diarrhea were given stool softeners for three days, the theory being that if they were faking to begin with the discomfort of having to defecate all the time was worse than submitting to their military duties. With such an approach to military medicine, Soviet units can be expected to have fewer "sick book riders" in their ranks than in Western armies. In most instances, reporting ill is not a good way to avoid military duties. If a soldier complains too often, or attempts to avoid duty or service with a false medical complaint, he can be charged with the crime of "malingering" and the punishment can be harsh. On balance, however, medical complaints and attempts to avoid service have not been signficant problems for the Soviet Army since 1967 when the Soviets established a nationwide system of premilitary training and physical screening.

Another factor that has reduced the problem of draft and duty avoidance has been the medical examiners' narrow view of psychiatric problems. A range of problems that might qualify an individual for rejection in Western armies are not acceptable in the Soviet Army. These problems include mild neurosis, anxiety, night sweats, or bed wetting, all of which are seen as signs of a lack of character or the result of a defective personality.

Finally, the Soviets reduce psychiatric exemptions from military service by distinguishing between individuals who can serve in combat units and those who can serve in noncombat duties. Based on the conscript's record and performance in premilitary training, a selection is made of those who may be better fit for more complex and technical assignments. These individuals also receive more extensive psychiatric screening, especially for such assignments as police units, missile units, and submarines. The Soviets believe that military manpower can be conserved by conscripting individuals with physical or even minor psychiatric problems and using them to good effect in noncombat duties. In addition, the Soviets maintain a large number of construction battalions to which almost anyone who meets even minimal standards can be assigned.

As a result of these practices, the military psychiatrist is not prominent in draft screening. Almost everyone is given a place in the military, even if this takes a little juggling. American intelligence estimates suggest that 92 percent of all conscripts called to military service eventually serve. No doubt much of this success is due to the Soviet view that psychiatrists are not allowed to interfere with the normal selection process to any great extent. The Soviets feel that too great an adherence to the Western experience would result in too great a rate of exemption from military service for psychiatric reasons.

SOVIET COMBAT MEDICAL DOCTRINE

In the first six months of World War II, the Soviets lost 2.4 million men killed and wounded, massive numbers which they were not equipped to handle. Their medical experience in the war taught them three lessons, all of which remain central to their medical combat doctrine today.

The first is that a medical system must be able to deal with the enormous number of casualties that occur in wars. The stress of war will make itself felt most clearly on the number of physical casualties which will be incurred and which can be saved through medical treatment. As in World War II, the Soviet medical corps does not treat psychiatric casualties seriously. Such casualties are relegated to the area of small psychiatry and are managed by political officers or within normal command channels. The Soviets would expect to endure great numbers of physical casualties in a nuclear war. The emphasis on casualties received renewed emphasis after 1967 when changes in Soviet battle doctrine forced a serious examination of the potential impact of nuclear weapons on casualty rates.

The second lesson is that the Soviets have completely integrated the entire civilian public health system into the military medical structure, so that most serious casualties can be expected to be treated at front-, army-, or district-level hospitals. Before going to war, they would first mobilize the entire civilian medical establishment and concript between eight and ten thousand doctors for military service. The integration of military and civilian medical facilities in an effort to mobilize the whole nation for war is a major characteristic of the army's combat medical structure.

Finally, casualties must be evacuated to rear areas for treatment rather than remain at the front. Defense Intelligence Agency studies on Soviet combat medical treatment reveal that the soldier is to be treated in the unit only to the extent needed to keep him alive so that he can be evacuated to the rear rather than holding him at regiment or battalion level and reintegrating him into his unit. Through this practice, the Soviets do not have to use a unit replacement system as do some of the Western armies. No real attempt is made to return wounded soldiers back to their original units.

Like the Americans, the Soviets replace individuals rather than units. In World War II, recovered wounded in the American Army did not normally return to their units, but were sent to replacement depots (not to be confused with the replacement battalions of the German Army) where they were individually sent to various units as the need arose. The Soviets have made one important change in this practice. Soviet combat doctrine requires that units be fought down to 30 to 40 percent strength before being replaced. Rather than refilling a unit with individual replacements, the Soviets would commit another unit to battle in its place, linking the replaced unit with the replacing unit, passing command to the new unit, and continuing the assault. Hence, a unit's membership and even command structure would keep changing as the battle raged. As a consequence, the Soviets would evacuate their wounded and have them recover at army, front, or district hospitals where they would then be reassembled at replacement depots. As these depots whole new units would be formed and then thrown into battle, so that the soldiers would not likely be returned to their original units.

Soviet historical experience has been reinforced by modern developments, namely, the likelihood of fighting on a nuclear battlefield. It has also been reinforced by the Soviet belief that chemical and biological agents which would be used in the next major war would generate tremendous numbers of casualties. Thus, the Soviet medical corps is configured first and foremost to deal with mass casualties by getting them out of the way so as not to hinder the offensive. This, in turn, is further supported by Soviet doctrine which requires a high tempo of battle in a continuous offensive to break the enemy's will. Because the Soviets also believe that a war in the West would be relatively short, perhaps lasting no more than ninety days, they would hope to gain victory quickly by getting the most out of their troops in a short period of time. In the Soviet view, there would be plenty of time, to treat the wounded and save what could be saved after their combat forces had defeated the enemy.

The relatively low priority given to treating rather than evacuating the wounded is suggested by the fact that medical supplies are given the lowest priority in the logistics train. Unlike Western armies, few organic vehicles in the division are dedicated to medical evacuation and almost none (as in the case of the Israeli Army) are dedicated to providing medical treatment. The Soviets are making only minimal efforts to use helicopters in a medical evacuation role, conditioned by the belief that the unarmed helicopter would be vulnerable to hostile fire in a modern war. Accordingly, evacuation of the wounded to regimental and division collection points would be carried out not by organic vehicles dedicated to the task, but by empty supply carriers. Trucks and Armored Personnel Carriers (APCs) would move to the front delivering Petroleum, Oil, and Lubricants (POL) and ammunition. On the way back to the rear resupply points, they would stop at regimental and divisional clearing stations to pick up the wounded and remove as many as possible of those tagged for evacuation, depending on the pace of battle. The major exception to this rule would be in the treatment of psychiatric casualties.

What is the impact of Soviet medical evacuation policies on psychiatric casualties? It must be remembered that the Soviets would use the same diagnostic and screening mechanisms they used in the World War II, which means that behavioral problems treated as true neuropsychiatric problems in the West would be treated as cowardice, lack of motivation, lack of will, improper training, or defective character by the Soviets. Accordingly, large numbers of neuropsychiatric casualties (by Western standards) would not be allowed in the medical evacuation chain at all, but would be handled in administrative or command channels by the unit commanders or the political officers. In the modern Soviet Army a political officer is assigned to every company, whereas in World War II one was assigned to each battalion. Hence, they have a much smaller number of personnel to deal with. One can reasonably expect that the screening of psychiatric casualties would be somewhat more thorough than it was in World War II or than it could be expected to be in Western armies. Based on this doctrine, Soviet medical and administrative personnel would likely refuse to recognize as legitimate any behavioral problem with no identifiable physical cause. The psychotic would, of course, be evacuated in the medical chain, but the use of conservative diagnostic definitions of psychiatric damage would go a long way in keeping neuropsychiatric cases out of the medical evacuation chain, as they did in World War II. For the most part, Soviet psychiatric casualties would be detained and treated in command channels or allowed to build up at the various medical clearing points where they would receive the lowest priority for evacuation and treatment.

Genuine neuropsychiatric casualties would be shunted into the normal medical evacuation chain and moved to the rear. Those soldiers with concussion, contusion, or other physiological problems associated with mental disturbance would be moved to at least division level and, in many cases, further rearward. They would be hospitalized at the neuropsychiatric ward of the army-level hospital for about two weeks to recover, and after recovery would be assigned to a replacement depot for further utilization. Western practice suggests that this might result in a greater number of deep neurosis casualties who might otherwise be turned around quickly. Once moved to the rear, secondary gain sets in and shock may deepen so that the soldier may require a much longer time to recover. On the other hand, if the Soviets can sustain the patient's belief that his problem is basically physiological in origin, once the physical aspects of the problem are addressed, recovery may be fairly rapid.

If Western models are correct, between 30 percent and 40 percent of soldiers exposed to battle in a future war could be expected to suffer a neuropsychiatric problem. The Soviet models offer different estimates, based on research using examples of shock effects found in natural disasters such as earthquakes, natural gas explosions, and large fires. Even in a nuclear battlezone, Soviet military psychiatrists do not expect any more than 10 percent of the casualties to result from genuine neuropsychiatric causes. With no way of treating neuropsychiatric casualties in lower echelon holding areas, the Soviet medical support system might find itself overwhelmed by the neuropsychiatric casualties. Yet, if their filtration systems, namely, the command channels, political officers, and clinical diagnostic definitions of a mental casualty operate as effectively as they did in World War II, then the number of psychiatric casualties who are evacuated back to division may well be lower than that in Western armies.

The propensity to evacuate soldiers to the rear for medical treatment has led to the use of drug therapies at the lower levels of the medical treatment system to stabilize shock casualties and then move them to the rear. No one can reasonably foresee to what extent this could lead to a degree of misdiagnosis so that they may end up placing neuropsychiatric patients in the medical chain that otherwise could be treated much more rapidly and effectively at the front. The emphasis on drug therapies to counter the physiological effects expected to result from nuclear shock and battle stress could create serious problems for the medical service by allowing some casualties to be evacuated that should not have been evacuated.

These circumstances raise a question as to the quality of medical personnel who would conduct the diagnostic screening of psychiatric casualties. In general, these personnel are not well equipped to perform this screening function. Many Soviet military psychiatrists believe that sanitors, feldshers, and even regimental surgeons may not have the training to recognize and diagnose neuropsychiatric casualties. This could lead to a number of additional problems.

First, soldiers suffering from true psychiatric problems could conceivably be turned over to the political officers and unit commanders without first receiving appropriate treatment. Second, large numbers of psychiatric casualties could be incorrectly diagnosed and screened and evacuated when they could be treated effectively and more rapidly at the lower echelon levels. The Soviet medical service has practically abandoned responsibility for all but the most severe neuropsychiatric symptomologies. As noted earlier, in practice, such cases are handled in command or political channels. Only those symptomologies accompanied by organic disruption can be adequately dealt with within the medical system.

Thus, soldiers with psychiatric problems unaccompanied by physical damage could easily be misdiagnosed, in which case they might be needlessly evacuated or forcibly returned to battle. The quality of medical training given to Soviet military medical personnel responsible for psychiatric casualties is a real problem indeed. The problem is evident even in Western armies as, for example, in the Israeli Defense Force (IDF). Although the IDF provides excellent doctors, psychiatrists, and psychologists in its field units for diagnostic screening and treatment of psychiatric casualties, during the 1982 war in Lebanon almost one-third, and perhaps as many as one-half, of the IDF's psychiatric casualty evacuations were misdiagnosed and needlessly evacuated to the rear.

Once a casualty reached division, he would be reexamined and a determination made as to whether to retain him at the division hospital or move him further to the rear. Regardless of the level at which the casualty would be retained, after two or three weeks special police units would make regular rounds of military hospitals and treatment sites, selecting soldiers sufficiently recovered from their wounds. These soldiers would then be sent to replacement depots where they would be assigned to new units and recommitted to battle. However else the Soviets handle the problem of evacuation of psychiatric casualties, the doctrine of expectancy would operate whether at lower or at higher levels. The point is to convince the Soviet soldier that a psychiatric disturbance is, in itself, not a legitimate cause for escaping one's military responsibilities. Even genuine psychiatric casualties would be expected to return to the fight. If the casualty was treated at the lower level, he might return within hours and certainly days. And even if evacuated to division, it is unlikely that he would spend more than four to six weeks before either returning to the fighting units or being discharged as a permanent casualty into the public health system. Those refusing to return would be forced to return.

PSYCHIATRIC CASUALTY SERVICING STRUCTURE

At front level, the Soviet Army maintains a complete psychiatric hospital with a director for psychiatric care and a special section for neuropsychiatric casualties. In addition, every military district has its own district hospital in which all medical specialties are available, including psychiatric care. The staff of the district hospital includes three or four neurologists and about the same number of psychiatrists. The Leningrad Military District Hospital, for example, has five neurologists and four psychiatrists on staff. These normally care for inpatients, whereas perhaps two additional doctors care for military outpatients. Both the front and district hospitals focus on neurologists. In general, the military regards neurologists as more valuable than psychiatrists because they can diagnose and treat the physical causes of brain disorders which are seen to be the root cause of psychiatric problems.

At army level, a small psychiatric ward accommodates up to forty beds. By and large, the psychiatric patient remains at army level for two weeks while undergoing treatment for minor psychiatric problems, three weeks if his problem is more serious, and no longer than six weeks if he has a truly serious problem. At the end of six weeks, the patient is either sent to a replacement depot or turned over to the civilian psychiatric establishment for further treatment. This discharge is normally accompanied by the assessment that the soldier can no longer be of any functional military use even in noncombat assignments.

The division level has the normal complement of battle surgeons and doctors but usually no psychiatrists or psychiatric wards. The division is seen as a combat fighting unit and is staffed mostly with medical surgical personnel who can deal with the common casualties of war. The Soviet Army has no equivalent of the division-level psychiatrist found in many Western armies. Equally important, it has no support staff of psychologists, social workers, or counselors which have become commonplace in Western armies, particularly in the Israeli and American armies. The problems handled by this staff are managed by the unit commander, his executive officer, or the political officer. At the divisional level, the political officer has a small staff of four to five persons, but normally they have more important tasks than dealing with psychiatric casualties.

At the regimental level, there is the normal medical staff comprised of a regimental surgeon and sometimes a neurologist, but, again, there are no psychiatrists or psychologists. The problems of small psychiatry are handled by the unit commander or the political officer. The same is true at battalion level except that no doctor is present. Medical treatment at battalion level is handled by the battalion feldsher, a trained physician's assistant. With regard to psychiatric casualties, medical personnel below division separate the truly serious neuropsychiatric cases from the less serious ones. In any future confrontation, the psychotic or those with psychiatric symptoms easily attributable to a physical cause would be evacuated to the next level for reexamination, treatment for a few days, or shipment further to the rear, depending on the severity of the problem. Minor cases would be turned over to command channels or the political officer to be dealt with on a "motivational basis." The first level at which a genuine neuropsychiatric casualty could be treated seriously would at army level. In the main, however, most instances of psychiatric disability would be treated functionally at the lower level by short periods of rest and returned to the line.

The training of medics, feldshers, and even doctors in psychiatric triage is almost nonexistent and well below that found in Western armies. The Soviets emphasize physical treatment over neuropsychiatric and neurotic reactions.

Unlike the American and Israeli armies, the Soviet Army has no psychiatric assistants for treating psychiatric casualties. Independent medical detachments under the authority of the Medical Department of the Chief of the Army Front may be sent to divisions to help out with medical problems, but none deals with psychiatric problems. For the most part they are nuclear, biological, and chemical teams, special surgical detachments, and even special equipment units, including specialists in the area of problems caused by extreme weather environments. There are no special psychiatric teams similar to those used by the Israeli Army or by the American Army in Vietnam. In the Soviet medical structure up to army level, there are no organic staffs to deal with neuropsychiatric cases as a special problem area. There are also no attached medical facilities that can be pressed into action. Although a small neuropsychiatric ward is located at the army-level hospital and an even larger ward at the front-level hospital, they are not usually staffed by psychiatrists. Most of the psychiatric work, as we have said, is done by neurologists.

Conversations with Soviet psychiatrists and battle surgeons suggest that the Soviet military is acutely aware that when certain kinds of physicians are within easy access of the troops, the troops tend to use them as a way of avoiding duty or battle. These Soviet physicians note rather high correlations between positioning neurologists near the troops and a tendency for the soldiers to show symptoms of nervous disorder. And they expect the same thing would happen if psychiatrists were made too accessible to soldiers. The Soviets also believe that the Western experience with psychiatric casualties in World War II, especially the American experience, was caused in large part by the presence of psychiatric diagnosticians too close to the troops and a lax set of diagnostic categories. As a consequence, the Soviets would not make psychiatric services readily available to the troops in a combat zone, feeling it to be self-defeating.

Not surprisingly, then, the Soviets do not have psychiatrists in their combat units and offer no psychological services at any level. In peacetime or in war, soldiers with problems cannot go to drug, alcohol, or family counselors, facilities that are common in most modern Western armies. They are required to deal with their problems by themselves or with the help of friends. As a rule, these problems seldom reach the political officer or the unit commander unless they disrupt the soldier's behavior, and at that time they are approached as disciplinary problems within the normal chain of command. Only rarely are they referred to medical personnel.

The political officer is a unique resource in the Soviet Army. Originally instituted to ensure the political loyalty of military commanders, the position has long since acquired more relevant functions. The Soviet Army is the only army in the world with an officer and small staff within combat units directly responsible for ensuring the morale, motivation, and fighting spirit of the soldier. In this sense, the political officer is an important adjunct to the commander. The Soviet commissar, although often denigrated in Western military literature, was often held in high esteem by soldiers in World War II. Combat histories of the Soviet Army show that the political officer was often the most motivated soldier in the unit and the most talented. Although many were also political hacks, by and large this situation has changed since the war's end. The Political Academy, which was founded prior to World War II, has been upgraded considerably, and most of the political officers today are college graduates. In addition, most have taken courses in psychology, if not psychiatry, to help them maintain morale and motivation. During World War II, the political officer was found only at battalion level or above. Today he is found at company level as well and, at some point in the future, he will likely be assigned to platoons.

Nicknamed "the priest" by the soldiers, the political officer is not usually sought out by the troops as a confidant and does not act as a counselor in the Western sense of the word. But it is his job to know what is going on among the troops in a unit, and little escapes his attention. Although the soldier is unlikely to seek him out, the political officer is quite likely to seek out the problem soldier if only to remind him of his responsibilities. In this sense, he can function as the first line of defense in locating and dealing with a soldier's psychological problems. Again, he handles these problems as a member of the command staff and not as a medical practitioner. However, the political officer's personal participation in battle and his presence on the frontline greatly increase his stature and authority in dealing with psychiatric problems. Soviet psychiatrists note that these conditions often make him more effective than trained psychiatrists who give advice safely from rear areas.

In peacetime, a soldier who is suffering from a psychiatric problem or who tries to commit suicide will almost always be sent to prison. He may, however, only be held in jail for a short time until a team of psychiatrists from the army- or front-level hospital can interview him and make a diagnosis. Even this type of examination requires a request from his commanding officer who, in making such a request, is admitting that he cannot handle the problem. As such, sending for a psychiatrist to examine a problem soldier is likely to occur only after the commander and the political officer have made repeated attempts to deal with the problem themselves. If an examination reveals that the problem is behavioral rather than physiological in origin, the soldier is usually returned to his commander for punishment or retained in prison. If, on the other hand, the soldier is truly mentally ill, he will usually be sent back to a rear area military hospital for treatment. If his problem can be cured or at least dealt with, he will then be returned to his unit to complete his military service and the time spent in the hospital will not generally be counted against his military enlistment. In short, only "bad time" must be made up.

The soldier with a diagnosis that cannot be managed by the military medical system is turned over to the public health system and discharged from the service. The rate of discharge for psychiatric problems in the Soviet Army in peacetime is very low. The Soviet authorities do not want to set a precedent of allowing individuals out of military service for this reason. Accordingly, soldiers with psychiatric problems that do not emanate from organic causes are dealt with very severely, and every effort is made to keep the soldier in military service even if he cannot be a useful member. For the Soviets, it is far more important to send the message to other soldiers that psychiatric debilitation will not be rewarded with release from military service than it is to ensure that the soldier receives adequate medical treatment.

PSYCHIATRIC TREATMENT

Soviet therapies for psychiatric patients have historically been based in biological theory, founded on the specific assumption that all behavior, including aberrant behavior, may be traced to organic disruption of brain functions. This approach has been characteristic of Russian psychiatry since before the turn of the century. With the partial rehabilitation of Soviet psychology as a separate discipline since the mid-1960s, other treatment methodologies, what the Soviets generically term socio-rehabilitative therapies, have been developed. By 1981 Soviet textbooks on the subject were calling each approach—the socio-rehabilitative and the biological—"equally important." Nonetheless, in most therapeutic environments it is the medical doctor, usually a neurologist or a psychiatrist, and not the psychologist, who generally oversees treatment. The biological approach is still dominant, and the mental hospitals are only rarely staffed by psychologists or other mental therapists. In those few situations where psychologists are allowed to conduct therapy, by law a medical doctor, often a neurologist, must be present or oversee the treatment. Nonbiological therapies are, in any case, regarded with suspicion and have yet to establish their validity in the eyes of the psychiatric establishment.

Basic biological therapies have been evident in Soviet military psychiatry at least since 1905 and have their parallel in the West. Some of the more common therapies include somatic, physical, active, narcotic sleep, insulin comatose, medical convulsive, and electroconvulsive therapies. With the rise of what the Soviets call the "pharmacological era of psychiatry,", many of these basic "biological shock" therapies have been replaced by drug therapies. Soviet psychiatrists apparently value drug intervention therapies and suggest that the use of psychopharmacological agents has greatly expanded the boundaries of therapeutic action. By the early 1970s, the drug revolution in the Soviet Union had taken full hold, and it has become a major feature in the treatment of psychiatric problems. For a list of major drugs used in Soviet psychiatric practice, along with the conditions for which they are prescribed, see Table 3.1.

The Soviets cite their own contributions to the development of psychopharmacological agents, but many of their claims are overstated. For the most part their most commonly used durgs are still imported, and most of the major advances were first made abroad, most notably in France, Germany, Hungary, and the United States. A number of Soviet drugs have been copied and given other names.

Despite the increase in the use of drug-related therapeutic techniques, control over therapies for treating combat shock or other mental problems in the military still resides with psychiatrists and neurologists. The concept of drug therapy has strengthened the idea of the organic origin of mental aberration and recommends itself as an excellent treatment therapy to psychiatrists because drugs work directly on the physiological functions of the brain. Soviet psychiatric specialists believe that mental illness has organic roots as a disease of the brain, a view that is not fully appreciated in the United States. From the Soviet perspective, psychology is a new and fundamentally untested discipline, and it continues to face strong opposition from the psychiatric establishment. As regards military psychiatrists, the basic diagnostic assumption remains that combat shock or any other mental aberration suffered by a soldier under fire is organic in origin and must be treated as such.

For the Soviets, psychotherapy remains a suspect area of study, a reputation that dates back to Stalinist days. Among psychotherapeutic

Table 3.1
Drugs Used by Soviet Military Psychiatrists in Treatment of Neurosis and Psychosis

For Psychosis:

  Anti-Psychotics:

Sedatives:	(Aminazine, Propazin, Levopromazine, Chlorprotixine, Reserpine, Leponex)
Selectives:	(Triftazin, Meterazine, Haloperidol, Carbidin, Pimozide)
Generals:	(Mazheptyl, Trisedyl)
Mood Elevators:	(Thyoridazine, Perphenazine, Frenolon, Fluorophenazine, Fluspiridine, Pimozide, Eglonyl)

  Anti-Depressants:

Sedatives:	(Amitriptylene, Surmontyl, Azaphine, Fluoracisin, Prothiaden, Osylidine, Pyrazidol)
Thymo-Analeptics:	(Imizine, Pertofran, Anafranil, Nortriptyline)
Stimulants:	(Iprazide, Nuredal, Benazide, Transamine, Nitrazepam)

For Reactive States/Neurosis:

  Tranquilizers:

Sedatives:	(Meprobamate, Amizyl, Chlordiazepoxide, Oxazepam, Nitrazepam, Phenazepam, Mebicar)

  Stimulators:

Minor Mood Elevators:	(Trioxazin, Diazepam, Medazepam)
Psycho-Stimulants:	(Pervitin, Meridil, Piridrol, Sydnocarb, Centrophinoxine, Pyriditol)

Source: G. Avrutskiy and A. A. Neduva, *Treatment of the Mentally Ill*, (Moscow: Meditsina, 1981), p. 56.

treatments are rational psychotherapy, auto-suggestion, suggestion in a state of wakefulness, autogenic training, hypnosis or hypnotherapy, and narco psychotherapy. In psychotherapy the use of psychotropic drugs is an essential component of the complex therapeutic action, and the value of such drugs is seen to lie basically in their ability to treat the organic causes of brain dysfunction. Thus, Soviet psychologists have made the appropriate bow in the direction of the dominant psychiatrists and their organic orientation toward psychiatric illness.

The Soviets have been engaged in clinical psychotherapy only since the mid-1970s, and, as a consequence, many of their treatment therapies still have major problems of acceptability. They have also had some difficulty in establishing the connection between therapies and success rates because they lack sufficient data bases to make statistical comparisons. Psychotherapy as practiced by Soviet psychologists is carefully controlled, for example, a public law guiding the use of psychotherapies is still in effect. This law, first promulgated by the People's Commissariat of Public Health, requires that psychotherapy must be conducted at all times in the presence of a psychiatrist or a physician. This decree was originally issued in 1926, but in Soviet textbooks it is still regarded as the main guideline for the use of psychotherapy in clinical situations.

In their treatment of stress, the Soviets make some use of folk and herbal medicines. Natural tranquilizers and stimulants such as valeriana, pantacrene, leonuria, ginseng, leuzeue, and eleuterococus continue to be used, although less so now than twenty years ago. Others, such as chloryl hydrate and cardiac bromide, are still widespread, as are calcium and magnesium IVs. These natural compounds are believed to have some advantages over alternative chemical compounds. They can be taken orally in droplet form; they do not overstimulate the patient; and they are not usually followed by exhaustion. In addition, natural stimulants are more easily absorbed by the body's system than are most synthetic compounds. On the battlefield, sanitors and feldshers carry medical kits that contain pills, liquids, and even injections of these natural compounds, along with the basic drugs for treating stress reactions. Although natural compounds are still much in evidence, the basic thrust of Soviet military psychiatry is toward developing synthetic drugs. Psychopharmacology is rapidly coming of age in the Soviet Union, and its developments tend to parallel those in the West.

With regard to treatments for syndromes specifically related to battle stress, the Soviets are trying to adopt the same diagnostic criteria used in the West. As noted earlier, the Ministry of Health has enforced the use of ICD-9 on the public health system in an effort to standardize diagnostic criteria. In general, the Soviets tend to use many of the same major diagnostic categories for defining problems related to battle-shock as they use in dealing with shock reactions resulting from other causes. In dealing with battle-shock reactions, psychiatrists use diagnostic categories that emphasize reactive states. They further subcategorize reactive states into acute shock reactions, depressive reactions, and reactive delirious psychosis. Other diagnostic categories related to battle-shock include neurosis, neurasthenia, hysterical neurosis, and hysterical psychosis. A diagnostic category, which is not common in the West but has a long history in the Soviet military, addresses those symptomatic psychoses resulting from infectious diseases. A relatively complete list of diagnostic categories, including a list of those frequently used in the West which are not used by Soviet psychiatrists, is presented in Tables 3.2 and 3.3.

Although a number of Soviet publications have discussed the use of

Table 3.2
Symptom Indicators Used by Soviet Military Psychiatrists to Diagnose Battle Neurosis and Psychosis

For Neurosis	For Psychosis
Irritability	Depression
Fatigue	Melancholia
Nervousness	Abulia
Insomnia	Apathy
Anxiety	Stupor
Phobia	Agitation
Low suppressed mood	Compulsion
Hypochondria	Delusion
Iatrogenia	Hallucination
Obsession	Denial of disease
	Depersonalization
	Extreme anxiety

Table 3.3
Common Terms Used in Western Military Psychiatry That Are Not Used by Soviet Military Psychiatrists

Post-Traumatic Stress Disorder

Anxiety Disorder

Battle Shock Syndrome

Neurotic Depression

drugs as a means of immunizing the soldier against battle stress, the available literature suggests that little information is useful to document the details of drug applications in this form. The Soviets are probably continuing research into the use of chemical agents which can help condition the soldier (as confirmed by conversations with present and former Soviet psychiatrists), but the exact details remain sketchy. Drug production and even experimentation with drug compounds are relatively new in the Soviet Union. In the recent past, the development of the Soviet drug industry lagged far behind that of the West, primarily because of the destruction caused by the war to the Russian homeland. Only in the last fifteen years has the Soviet Union begun to catch up with the West in drug production. But in terms of the variety and purity of drug production, the Soviet drug industry is still behind.

Interviews with Soviet psychiatrists as well as medical doctors and pharmacologists reveal that their drug applications are plagued by poor quality of drug purity and refinement. The drug industry has not yet reached the same level of manufacturing precision as in the West; thus, drugs often produce a number of unwanted and paradoxical side-effects. As a consequence, many of the tranquilizers and stimulants used in the Soviet Union are imported, with West Germany and France the most common sources from the West, and East Germany and Hungary the prime sources from Eastern Europe. As mentioned earlier, by Western standards the Soviet drug industry is still relatively primitive. But the clinical application of drugs is quite advanced and, at least in terms of the time required to get a new drug into the clinical marketplace, much faster than in the United States.

Soviet technical literature has high praise for the potential uses of psychostimulators and tranquilizers. It is not surprising that the Soviets are seriously exploring drugs as a mechanism for conditioning the soldier against stress, given their physiological assumptions as explanations for human behavior.

In terms of psychostimulants, Soviet technical literature reveals that the following positive effects can be used to aid the soldier in coping with battle stress: (1) activation of intellectual activity, which can help process information; (2) acceleration of the processes of thinking and speaking; (3) mild euphoria; (4) increased activity and temporary elimination of fatigue; and (5) stimulation of altertness and decrease in appetite. Chemical stimulants include not only artificial compounds, but also such natural stimulants as caffeine, alcohol, and extract of magnolia vine.

Despite the interest in the military applications of psychostimulants and tranquilizers, a survey of Soviet medical literature during a twenty-year period reveals only a handful of publicized applications of research dealing with military uses for drugs and battlefield behavior. Even the few studies that are available are relatively recent. More recent still is the research on improving the soldier's physical performance through drugs and auto-suggestion. For years the Soviets have given preeminence to political training and other forms of conditioning to "steel the will" of the soldier against stress. Only within the last decade or so has there been any work moving beyond this approach to actual clinical applications.

A small list of drugs that appear in Soviet medical literature have military applications. The degree of military application, however, remains in question. The Soviets are apparently still in the testing stages and are using them essentially in clinical research settings. There is no hard evidence of any widespread practical applications for using psychostimulants and other drugs in battle.

Some of the drugs covered in the technical literature that have potential military applications include Phenamine (amphetamine sulfate) which was used in World War II. This drug may have been the first psychostimulant used by the Soviets to increase battlefield performance, and it may still be in use today. It produces a short-term burst of energy, but it is often accompanied by highly paradoxical side-effects and causes exhaustion. Another drug, Penatine, a combination of phenamine and nicotine, is also used as a stimulant. In 1969 it was used in a series of small experiments with artillery gunners in order to determine how long gunners could continue to fire while under the influence of the stimulant. Ostensibly, its effects are milder than phenamine alone without producing addiction or severe exhaustion.

A third drug is Syndocarb, a general but strong stimulant that may be somewhat better than Amphetamine. Because it is a stronger compound, the Soviets feel it can be more easily targeted against specific symptoms. Its impact on the organism develops more gradually than Amphetamine, so that there is no "rush" of excitement, and it is longer lasting in its effects. Syndocarb also seems to produce neither euphoria nor motor excitation, and, apparently, has only limited side-effects such as muscle weakness or inability to sleep.

Two other Soviet drugs are Phenaput and Trioxizine. Phenaput is a broad spectrum tranquilizer which is probably not akin to valium or any other benzodiazephine and is a derivative of GABA. Trioxizine is also a tranquilizer with identifiable properties like librium. Phenaput was used in military experiments as early as 1970 by L. I. Spivak before he became chief of the Department of Psychiatry at the Kirov Military Medical Academy. In the experiments, an attempt was made to reduce stress among paratroopers and riflemen by administering the drug to these soldiers over a twenty-day period and measuring the differences in their ability to hit rifle targets. Phenaput may also be used to reduce fear and extend motor activity. The Soviets used this drug during the American-Soviet space link-up with Soyuz.

In assessing the effectiveness of drug applications as a means of immunizing and controlling stress, we may state that, although the Soviets will pursue this line of research in the years ahead, at present their research is probably no further advanced than that of the West. In fact, they may be considerably behind Western research efforts. More importantly, whatever military applications the Soviets may have developed have been restricted to small research projects. There is no evidence of widespread use of either tranquilizers or psychostimulants as preventatives or as immunizers of stress within the military. In light of the physiological orientation of Soviet military psychiatry, they will likely continue to put significant effort into finding chemical means to increase the efficiency of the physiological mechanisms which they see as conditioning human behavior.

Soviet military psychiatry holds that reactive states are caused by short-term traumatic impacts on the soldier. Trauma refers exclusively to physical injury, and not, as in the United States, to a nonphysical impact that might produce psychological reactions. The onset of a reactive state is very rapid and is, therefore, distinguished from the effects of long-term battle fatigue. Reactive states can set in within hours or even minutes of exposure to trauma. In the Soviet view psychotic reactions are directly related to the traumatic event and are not a mechanism for triggering deeper psychological problems. In addition, the reversibility of a psychotic reaction is in direct proportion to the degree and impact of the initial trauma. This view fits well with the traditional notion that trauma acts primarily to disrupt the physiology of the brain by disordering the conditioned reflexes of the second signal system.

SOVIET MILITARY PSYCHIATRY

The Soviets maintain that their view of trauma-induced psychosis as being caused by a disruption of brain function is realistic. They define reactive states as having certain characteristics, the first of which is functionality. The reactive state is regarded as a functional response to stress which allows the soldier to escape from battle or to close off some horror he may have witnessed. Accordingly, the Soviets understand the problem of secondary gain. They understand that a soldier "gains" or profits from remaining in his reactive state. As a way of approaching treatment, they make every effort to demonstrate to the soldier, either through traumatic therapy or threats of punishment, that this gain will not be tolerated.

A second characteristic of reactive states is their reversibility and temporary nature, a view that is directly deducible from the Soviet assumption that the brain learns by conditioned response. The objective of treatment is to recondition the brain or shock it back into its normal pattern of operation. Once the trauma abates and the brain returns to working normally again, the reactive state should dissipate. In short, if brain patterns have been disordered by trauma, the removal of the trauma—or the infliction of a stronger stimulus—ought to break the psychosis. There is no question of psychosis lingering in the absence of trauma, in the sense that it results from deeper psychological problems which the trauma happened to bring to the surface.

A third characteristic of reactive states is their essentially nonpsychogenic aspect. That is, reactive states do not result from long standing psychological problems, but rather are a specific and temporary response to traumatic conditions which the organism has suffered. The removal of the soldier from these conditions is often sufficient to reverse the syndrome.

Soviet military psychiatrists clinically distinguish three types of affective battle reactions: acute affective shock, depressive psychogenic shock, and reactive delirious psychosis. In the first type, acute affective shock, the onset of the reactive state is very rapid and takes many forms, including paralysis, blindness, and surdomutism. Rarely will acute reactions produce a psychogenic stupor, but they will occur from time to time. In general, stupor is placed in the category of depressive reactions. With regard to treatment, the individual is immediately isolated from the traumatic event and moved out of the risk zone. He is also insulated from the rest of the members of his unit in order to prevent any contagion, although the contagion effect is denied any validity in Soviet psychiatric theory. If necessary, the soldier is immobilized with restraints. Drugs are administered immediately to stabilize the patient. Frequent heavy-impact doses, as much as 100 to 150 milligrams, are given by injection on the spot until the sedative effect takes hold. The drugs of choice to treat acute affective shock are Phenazapen, Phenazepam, Ilenium, Siduzin, and Amitriptylene, all of which are strong tranquilizers. After the patient has been sedated, other tranquilizing doses are administered to sustain the sedated condition. These less powerful but sustaining compounds include Aminazine, Tisercin, and Chloprotixine. These are also administered in relatively high doses until the patient has recovered.

The Soviets find that the most common manifestation of reactive psychosis is what they call depressive reactions. Here they recommend an intense therapy utilizing Amitriptylene, an antidepressant. Again the practice is to administer heavy initial doses to prevent a deepening of the depression. They distinguish between types of depression and prescribe different degrees of drug doses to deal with them. In general, however, a true psychotic depression is usually treated with very high doses of Ampriptylene, Melipramine, and Pyrazdol. Shallow depression seems to respond fairly well to high doses of Azaphen.

Reactive delirious psychosis, a severe reactive depression accompanied by strong physiological symptoms, is referred to as a "tightened reactive state" by Soviet psychiatrists. It is characterized by such extreme symptoms as delirium of pursuit, auditory hallucinations, surdomutism, and a complete disassociation from reality. In treating this condition, the Soviets have made use of neuroliptics such as Triftazin, Perheneazine, and Trisedil. They recognize the validity of a number of psychotraumatizing situations encountered in battle. These situations can cause extreme pyschomotor excitation in the soldier which may last for several hours. The symptoms include sensory delirium, false perceptions, and strong affective fear. Soviet psychiatrists suggest that strong and immediate treatment be rendered to deal with these symptoms before the syndrome can gain a strong hold on the individual. Their experience suggests that the rapidity of treatment is fundamental to reversing the reaction. Reactive delirious psychosis is treated like cases of acute shock, and the therapy of choice is to administer strong neuroliptics with sedative effects. Some more commonly prescribed drugs used in these cases include Aminazine, Levopromozene,

Chrlophophysine, and Tryphotizine, all given intramuscularly and in high dosages. In specific cases of extreme psychomotor excitation resulting from trauma the use of Aminezene and Levopromozine at 25 to 50 milligrams a day by injection is recommended. Also used is a 2 percent solution of Dimedrol, a 25 percent solution of Magnesium Sulphate, or a solution of Barbamyl in combination with a 10 percent solution of Glucanated Calcium and 10 percent Calcium Chloride administered intravenously. In the treatment of hysterical stupor, the use of psychomotor stimulants is prescribed using Syndocarb at 30 to 40 milligrams a day accompanied by a mild tranquilizer.

Soviet military psychiatrists stress that reactive psychosis is strongly associated with battle stress. Not that they are unaware that there are other kinds of reactions to battle-shock. But the primary emphasis seems to be on dealing with reactive psychosis, and the reason is clear enough. If one takes the view that the soldier's behavior is totally a function of the organic operations of the brain and that any disruption of brain function will produce physiological symptoms (and vice versa), then the focus on the strong physiological symptoms that accompany reactive psychosis is logical. It is here that the soldier will most commonly manifest the kinds of problems that will have the greatest effect on the combat unit. More importantly, reactive psychosis is accompanied by clear physiological disruptions and symptomology that facilitate diagnosis by a psychiatrist rather than a battle surgeon. Accordingly, it is not surprising that the Soviets tend to emphasize reactive states in their treatment of battle stress. It is this combination of a physiological and psychiatric problem that Soviet psychiatrists can best manage, considering their biological assumptions about the roots of human behavior.

Soviet psychiatrists are not trained to deal with psychiatric problems that have no clear accompanying physiological symptoms and that, in the West, may be regarded as originating purely in the emotions. In the Soviet view, as already stated, such problems are not recognized as legitimate psychiatric problems at all but as problems of "small psychiatry." But in reactive psychosis one finds the precise case for which the Soviet psychiatrist is so well trained, namely, a psychiatric disturbance caused by a physiological trauma that manifests itself in external symptoms that can be managed directly, usually through drug therapy affecting the organic operations of the brain. It is hardly surprising, then, that Soviet military psychiatrists concentrate on reactive psychosis as the most important form of neuropsychiatric breakdown with which they would have to deal in future wars.

Although Soviet military psychiatrists recognize a wide range of other battle-shock reactions, they do not seem to spend much time and effort in treating them. In the treatment of neurosis, for example, which they see as a consequence of fear and anxiety, Soviet psychiatrists are likely to regard it as a minor problem and treat it with short-term tranquilizer therapy. Except when the neurosis is deep and debilitating, they will frequently define the condition as one appropriate to small psychiatry to be handled appropriately outside medical channels. In treating neurosis, vegeostabilizers are used to break down the physiological disruptions in the organism which are the cause of fear and anxiety. In dealing with neurasthenia, Soviet psychiatrists seem to take the condition only slightly more seriously. Neurasthenia takes the form of weakness, exhaustion, increased reduction of mental and physical efficiency, transitions of mood, and an inability to focus and process information. These symptoms are regarded as hypostenic as opposed to hyperstenic forms of neurasthenia. The major treatment recommended is tranquilizer therapy to break the organic reaction patterns—what the Soviets call vegetative disruption of autonomic nervous system patterns. In the hyperstenic forms of neurasthenia (an interesting diagnosis in itself), the syndrome is characterized by an extreme form of excitation. Once again tranquilizing drugs are recommended, including Meprobamate, Emisile, Elinium, Trapazine, and Phenazecom. In its hypostenic forms, neurasthenia is treated with antidepressant drugs and stimulants including Trioxizine, Sougexin, and the psychostimulants Syndocarb and Sindophine. The Soviets emphasize that, as with other problems related to battle stress, the treatment of neurasthenia should begin as quickly as possible. They emphasize that the possibility of psychological dependence on drugs should also be monitored.

Soviet psychiatrists have achieved some success in the treatment of asthenic states through the use of a new class of drugs called "nootropes." While little has been published in Soviet literature about this new class of drugs, it is believed to work basically by effecting the metabolism of the cells of the brain. Examples are Iminalon and Ancebol. Only sparse information about the efficacy of these drugs or their chemical composition is available, but one Soviet pharmacologist noted that they were invented in Japan as GABA derivatives and are widely used in Europe where they are manufactured under license.

Soviet military psychiatrists also recognize three other categories of battle-shock reactions: hysterical neurosis, hysteria, and pyschasthenia. Hysterical neurosis is characterized by short-term, reversible, and pyschogenically nonpsychotic disorders. Examples of this condition are temporary mutism, asthasia, abasia, hysterical fits, and weeping. The specific conditions that separate hysterical neurosis from reactive psychosis are unclear except that one distinguishing factor seems to be the rapidity with which the patient responds to treatment. Thus, the initial treatments for dealing with hysterical neurosis are the traditional ones (used in World War I by almost all armies) of slapping or shaking the soldier, shouting, causing pain, immersion in cold water, or any other means of causing a shock to the patient in order to bring him out of his condition. More modern treatments follow if the syndrome cannot be broken in the traditional manner. These treatments require the administration of drugs such as Elinium and Phynazepam by injection.

Another category, hysteria, is defined as affective instability expressed in behavior and is generally characterized by the same symptoms as hysterical neurosis, although not as deeply. The treatment of choice is either shock or tranquilizers. A third category, psychasthenia, is characterized by an alarming overanxiousness and uncertainty about one's ability and surroundings, usually accompanied by lowered moods. The use of psychostimulators is indicated in the treatment of this condition.

In addition, the Soviets have identified a psychiatric disruption that is organically based and that seems to be almost absent from American literature. This is the psychiatric, often psychotic, reaction to poisoning or infectious disease, a condition called exogenic symptomatic psychosis which the Soviets believe is based in the patient's disrupted physiology. Soviet military psychiatrists identify five basic types of symptomatic psychosis: delirium, epileptic excitation, twilight states, confusion, and hallucinations. Inasmuch as armies throughout history have almost always suffered more casualties from disease than from enemy fire, the focus on mental aberrations caused by disease processes probably has a long history in Soviet military medicine. Moreover, it is the kind of problem that would find a ready audience within

Soviet psychiatry given its biological assumptions about human behavior. Because organic patterns may be disrupted not only by battle-shock but also by disease, fever, and viruses, the Soviet military psychiatrist is comfortable in dealing with the psychiatric effects of infectious diseases.

Soviet military medical literature emphasizes treatment of mental disruptions caused by the external environment. The impact of extreme heat and cold on the soldier's ability to maintain the mental strength to continue the battle has been closely studied. This direction of study is only moderately evident in American military psychiatry, and, where it is, it is not reflected in the research of psychiatrists as much as in the work of battle surgeons. In the Soviet case, one again encounters the tendency to join the medical doctor and the psychiatrist at the point of common origin, where the physiological disruption of the brain produces behavioral aberrations.

FUTURE DIRECTIONS

With regard to psychiatry, future research and field applications will likely continue to focus on the "revolution in psychopharmacology," that is, on the utilization of drugs both to prevent and to treat psychiatric illnesses resulting from combat stress. It is highly unlikely that Soviet military psychiatry will abandon its basic assumptions, if for no other reason than that they seem to have worked well during World War II. The Soviets believe their applications of combat psychiatry have already proven far superior to those of the West insofar as they helped preserve their manpower base during the Great Patriotic War. They fully expect these same assumptions to prove effective in any future encounter.

Soviet psychiatry will probably remain essentially as it has been for the last twenty years and is unlikely to produce any revolutionary developments. Characteristically, the Russians are proceeding gradually, only slowly incorporating incremental changes. Yet, it must be said that, although Soviet psychiatry, especially in relation to its diagnosis and treatment of illnesses related to battle stress, accepts premises that are regarded as highly questionable in the United States, in practice their system seems to work fairly well in dealing with psychiatric casualties. No one can deny that in World War II the Soviets had a much lower rate of manpower loss resulting from psychiatric problems than did most Allied armies, particularly the United States. Furthermore, the political structure reinforces the diagnostic categories and treatment mechanisms used by the military psychiatric establishment. Interestingly, they are essentially the same diagnostic criteria and treatments used by Western armies during World War I.

Men under stress often manifest the very symptoms that are most readily recognized by the diagnostic categories used by medical examiners to decide if the soldier is to be removed from stressful situations. Accordingly, if a severe case of the "war tremors" is sufficient to permit a soldier to escape the stress of battle, then it comes as no surprise that soldiers tend to develop precisely this condition when the horrors of war increase. In the Soviet case, if reactive psychosis is what is required to obtain relief from battle, then Soviet soldiers will likely develop reactive psychosis. Thus, the values of the military subculture may well play a much larger role in determining combat reactions. When treatments for combat reactions are harsh, this in itself may also affect the frequency with which psychiatric breakdown occurs. The Soviets, believing this to be the case, have designed their theory and practice of combat psychiatry accordingly.

When theory becomes institutionalized as structure and power, theoretical propositions and analytical categories risk becoming self-fulfilling prophecies. In the realm of things psychic, perhaps what ultimately matters most are the values and expectations that men have of themselves and their peers. These factors, more than any others, may be the most important determinants of behavior under fire. Certainly the Soviets seem to think this is the case, and their military psychiatry will probably continue to reflect this view until events prove them wrong.

REFERENCES

Dupuy, T. R. (1970). *The encyclopedia of military history*. New York: Harper & Row.

Ginzberg, Eli. (1959). *The lost divisions*. New York: Columbia University Press.

4

Military Psychiatry in the German Army

ROBERT SCHNEIDER

Combat stress reaction (CSR) refers to a transient anxiety reaction in the soldier, which leads to his temporary incapacitation and inability to continue fighting for some period of time. Most of the military, historical, and medical analyses of the Wehrmacht's performance in World War II conclude that the German soldier did not experience serious problems owing to stress breakdown of soldiers (Van Creveld, 1983). The reasons are rooted in the exceptional quality of small-unit military leadership in the German Army and the high degree of social cohesion manifested by German military units.

This position suggests that the German Army is the only force in modern memory that has not suffered serious problems of stress reaction among its soldiers in combat. Yet, CSR has been a source of significant and continued manpower loss to virtually every other army, requiring medical and command attention for both prevention and treatment. Studies of the German Army in World War II indicate that combat stress reactions were, in fact, a serious problem for the Wehrmacht, but certain societal forces present in prewar Germany so affected military psychiatric practice as to almost preclude German psy-

---

The views of the author do not purport to reflect the positions of the department of the army or the department of defense (Para 4-3, AR-360-5).

chiatrists from acknowledging the possibility of CSR. Thus, previous analyses have concluded that the Germans had few problems in this area simply because they have accepted the distorted German view concerning this problem.

The subject is of more than mere historical interest. A number of current military writers have emphasized the potential for profound command and manpower problems resulting from stress breakdown on the modern battlefield (Belenky, Jones, and Newhouse, 1981; Ingraham and Manning, 1980; Schneider and Luscomb, 1983). The Israeli Defense Force, a very well-led and highly cohesive military force, has experienced considerable numbers of CSR casualties in its recent wars (Belenky, Noy, and Soloman, 1985; Noy, 1982; Rock and Schneider, 1984). The Israeli experience suggests, however, that the findings and doctrines developed by other armies are indeed useful for preventing and treating the problem. Chief among these is the importance of strong unit cohesion and well-trained combat leadership. Thus, if the Wehrmacht performed as well in this area as other analysts have suggested, then it is worthwhile to investigate the quality and development of leadership and unit cohesion manifested by that army. If, on the other hand, the Wehrmacht did suffer serious rates of CSR, then documenting this fact would fill an important gap in our historical military knowledge. It would also provide additional evidence that CSR cannot be prevented *in toto* in even the best of armies.

Obtaining data concerning CSR in the Wehrmacht has proved quite difficult. Little is known about the phenomenon during World War II, and what is available is limited and written almost exclusively in German. Furthermore, during 1939–1945, relatively little was published about German military medicine in general, and even less about military psychiatry. Finally, the available material tends to indicate that stress reactions were not a serious problem for the Wehrmacht in terms of numbers of soldiers lost to combat or of impact on medical resources. Yet, it is difficult to accept this position, for it would mean that the German Army, alone among modern armies exposed to combat, suffered few such casualties. The solution was to interview soldiers and psychiatrists who served in the Wehrmacht with first-hand knowledge of the German soldier in combat.

My first interviews, with several psychiatrists who had served in the Wehrmacht, proved of little help to my thesis, for they stated that the Wehrmacht did not suffer CSR, for the various reasons which I will discuss below. But in interviews with two individuals who had served as noncommissioned officers (NCOs), one described seeing a soldier who had been hanged, with a sign around his neck reading "I was a coward." But the dead soldier had an Iron Cross medal on his chest, a medal awarded for valor in combat; if this soldier was a coward, he had clearly not always been so. He also described soldiers who after days of fighting quit, withdrawing and refusing to talk or go on. The second interviewee described a soldier who would get a headache every time he was ordered into his tank. The headaches were so severe that he could not fight. These first-hand accounts suggested that perhaps other cases had manifested similar symptoms. My investigation eventually led me to the German Military Archives, which provided an overwhelming amount of data on medical practice in World War II. Generally, this material revealed that, in spite of the fact that many reported CSR was not a problem, it was frequently mentioned and entire conferences were devoted to it. Difficulties of agreeing on a diagnosis, labeling, and a treatment dominated the topics of psychiatric meetings throughout the war. These difficulties were exacerbated by certain societal influences affecting medical practice. Among these influences were advances in the understanding of diseases and the rise of the National Socialist (NAZI) party to power in Germany.

In order to understand the medical problem of recognizing and treating CSR, one must first comprehend the variety of forms the reaction can take. Soldiers afflicted manifest a variety of somatic complaints, ranging from body pains to headaches to gastrointestinal upset. CSR can also manifest itself as sleep disturbance, psychomotor disturbance, or depression, and can include venereal disease, frostbite, self-inflicted wounds, and antisocial behavior. Although there is much overlap, Baron et al. (1983) demonstrate that in each war a certain cluster of symptoms seems to dominate. As this cluster changes with each war, early recognition is often made difficult for an army. The U.S. Army, for example, was not prepared to treat stress casualties at the outset of World War II, even though it had developed a successful treatment in World War I (Glass, 1954).

CSR can usually be reversed with proper treatment. It occurs in soldiers both directly or indirectly exposed to combat, and it is positively related to the intensity and duration of exposure to combat. Other characteristics of the battle, such as type of weapons, time (night or day), and pace of movement, affect the rates of soldier breakdown, as do a number of organizational and group characteristics, such as morale, cohesion, and quality of leadership (Glass, 1955). All soldiers are at risk for CSR, because exposure to sufficient stress will ultimately result in virtually every soldier becoming a stress casualty (Beebe and Appel, 1958). Proper treatment comprises early, rapid, but simple therapies (abreaction and rest, called "immediacy" and "simplicity"), close to the front (called "proximity"). Treating the casualty as a soldier (rather than as a patient) to foster the idea that he will soon return to duty (called "expectancy") has historically led to a recovery rate of about 75 percent within seventy-two hours. About 25 percent of the number of wounded patients can be expected to manifest stress breakdown; such casualties, therefore, comprise a considerable pool of potentially recoverable manpower. There is no personality or "behavioral weakness" that predisposes a soldier to breakdown in combat.

Treatment of the stress casualty is considered a medical problem, although prevention of CSR is generally regarded as a command or leadership issue. The relationship of these two areas (medicine and leadership) in German society and the military prior to World War II provides a starting point to examine and understand CSR in the Wehrmacht. The examination begins with an explanation of certain historical and political influences on medicine in Germany prior to the war, as well as the German view of leadership.

In the early part of this century, psychiatry was committed to finding an organic basis for dysfunctional behavior. This probably reflected advances in other fields of medicine, such as physiology, neurology, and biochemistry which were increasingly able to identify the causes and agents of disease and maldevelopment. Severe mental problems were especially thought to be due to organic causes and, therefore, consumed the most attention of psychiatric practitioners (Albee, 1985). As medicine advanced and the organic cause of each disease was discovered, a description and classification followed shortly. Classifiers of psychiatric "disease," therefore, focused on severe problems like paresis, delirium tremens, schizophrenia, and manic-depressive psychosis, each of which was believed to have an organic basis.

Western combat psychiatry during World War I reflected the influence of this orientation. Stress breakdown in battle was labeled shell shock. This label reflected the early belief that it was due to internal damage to the brain, caused by the shock of nearby explosions. But in most cases of CSR, no obvious organic damage (such as ruptured eardrums) could be demonstrated. Furthermore, internal damage to the brain could not usually be found on autopsy. At first, the influence of the organic explanation for disease was strong enough to override these facts. Organic damage or changes in the brain were presumed to be so small that the available means could not dicern them. The organic explanation for abnormal behavior was indeed persistent in psychiatry, and this influence was equally strong on both sides of the Atlantic.

The major force countering this explanation was probably the work of Sigmund Freud. Focusing on the more common neuroses such as phobia, hypochondriasis, and hysteria, Freud revised diagnostic thinking. His therapy centered on the role of the subconscious mind, essentially refuting the role of organic causation in the most frequent forms of mental "disease." One important outcome of his approach was that understanding the cause of psychiatric problems was no longer very simple, and treating them required psychotherapy which often stretched to months or years. As a theory and treatment that countermanded prevailing medical belief, it naturally met strong resistance.

At the same time, several factors existed in Germany that served to reduce the impact or acceptance of the Freudian explanation of behavior even further. First, the NAZI movement was gaining strength and Germany was beginning to prepare for war. This factor had several implications for the practice of psychiatry. The Nazi party embraced the idea of the "human factor" as a challenge to materialism, liberalism, and Marxism. The human factor included racial and national character, practicality, health, and comradeship (Madej, 1978). These, in combination with "strength of will," formed part of the basis of the Nazi view of how Germany could fight an enemy that had superior numbers. The human factor could contribute to increased productivity as well as decreased conflict between management and labor (Cocks, 1985). Training by industrial psychologists was an important part of the effort to build on the human factor. Although the contributions of these psychologists were not in the area of direct patient treatment, they did enjoy an increase in status at the apparent expense of psychiatry.

Second, psychiatrists were competing with psychologists to limit the practice of psychology (Cocks, 1985). This effort initially involved preventing psychologists from the practice of psychoanalysis (it was to be reserved for physicians) altogether. When this failed, control of psychologists' training (physicians had to train psychologists to practice psychotherapy) and practice (psychologists could only practice psychotherapy under the direction of a psychiatrist) was sought. This move dissipated their influence as psychologists increased their influence in other areas (e.g., industrial psychology and education), while psychiatrists concentrated on discrediting psychology rather than expanding their own functions and applications.

Third, Freud, the father of psychotherapy, was Jewish. As a result, his work was suspect and in some quarters reviled (Cocks, 1985). This factor alone might have been enough to discredit the psychoanalytic explanation of dysfunctional behavior in Nazi Germany. But there were other influences as well. In terms of the military, with the Nazi emphasis on will and character, the concept of an emotionally maladjusted soldier did not sit well. There was no room for the subconscious in the "human factor." There was a practical matter to consider as well. With a population of only about 80 million, German military planners recognized that they needed every available soldier. A therapy that could take weeks or months to return a soldier to duty was not acceptable. Thus, long-term psychotherapy was unacceptable not only for political reasons, but also for practical reasons.

These factors made themselves felt in spite of the German experience in World War I when hysterical reactions to combat were quite common. They took the form of paralysis and trembling, which rendered the soldier incapable of further action. The number of soldiers affected with this condition is not known but must have been high. Treatment followed a French technique called "torpillage"—the application of a painful electric shock to the paralyzed limb. The cure rate for this treatment was high, although the magnitude of the problem was referred to as "very serious" in guidelines for psychiatric support for the coming war (*Allgemeine Richtlinien*, 1939).

In terms of military psychiatry, these factors had several effects. Military medical planning did not include recognition or treatment of psychogenic problems or any dysfunctional behavior that would be recognized as CSR today. The human factor was under the control of the military leader, who was responsible for ensuring that the German ideal of the strong committed soldier be met in his unit. The psychiatrist or psychologist was used for consultation purposes to provide advice on how to maximize the human factor in training soldiers or in personnel selection. Breakdown in combat was to be considered as the result of either an organic cause (like shell shock in the earlier war) or the weak character of the affected soldier. Organic problems could (and should) be treated by the psychiatrist, but under the influence of the National Socialists, other behavioral problems could not. The other behavioral problems (frequently called "cowardice") were attributed to "weak wills," or other failures to properly train and indoctrinate the soldier.

Once behavioral problems occurred, they were clearly under the purview of military leadership rather than medical or psychiatric officers. It was, therefore, a leadership responsibility to prevent and treat dysfunctional behavior. Naturally, treatment began with an examination by a psychiatrist, who had first to determine whether an organic problem was present. Organic problems included outright psychosis as well as medical problems of a known organic basis (such as delirium tremens). Mental retardation was also a frequent diagnosis. Soldiers with problems that the psychiatrist could not attribute to an organic cause were "treated" via other channels to increase their will to serve. Such treatment included assignment to a special work battalion where discipline was emphasized or eventual assignment to a concentration camp. A considerable number of Wehrmacht medical documents deal with the problems of malingering and cowardice. Many cases of soldier breakdown were considered to be due to cowardice, a viewpoint consistent with the Nazi view of the German soldier as brave and strong. The Nazis recognized the presence of Communists and other "undesirable" types, and the psychiatrist was expected to identify them for elimination from the service.

The Wehrmacht took the practice of leadership quite seriously. Although the influence of psychiatrists, especially those who practiced psychoanalysis, had been reduced, psychiatrists retained a strong role in the military. They served as consultants to major commanders on a number of soldier-related issues, including methods of training, amount of training, morale building, and even diet. An examination of original Wehrmacht medical documents shows that many (perhaps most) major decisions concerning the soldier's health and welfare were made with the consultation of a psychiatrist. Cocks (1985) provides a concise summary of this influence:

The proper combination of worker and machine, for one thing, rested on an understanding of the human psyche, an accurate assessment rendered more attractive to the Nazis through its trust in the qualitative powers of the German will over and above the harder and more tangible coordinates of technology and numbers (p 200).

Psychologists were not included in military command consultations; their use was apparently limited to selection and basic training. Psychiatrists were also used as a kind of "ombudsman" who would investigate the cause of problems in the case of unit-wide complaints. The Wehrmacht used every approach to ensure that its men were taken care of, and the psychiatrist could be very helpful in this task.

As the Wehrmacht prepared for war, there was no developed official medical doctrine for the treatment of CSR. Logically, such a doctrine was not necessary inasmuch as breakdown in battle was not a medical problem. Once the soldier left the training base, prevention was also a leadership problem. Medical practitioners were, therefore, not trained or prepared to recognize CSR if it occurred. But this naturally followed the belief that breakdown would not occur. German medicine shared the view of its society: Leadership and will would provide the advantage the army needed. The German soldier had the "human factor" in his favor.

This view of soldier resistance emerged clearly in an interview with a German military psychiatrist, Dr. Rudolf Brickenstein, a junior psychiatrist in the Wehrmacht during the war. His specific interest was in suicide, an area that should have exposed him to the problems of stress in battle. By 1982, he had risen to the position of highest ranking psychiatrist in the Bundeswehr. In an interview, he stated that there were no serious problems due to stress breakdown among German soldiers, because the high quality of Wehrmacht leadership prevented it. It should be pointed out here that in the interviews it was difficult to agree on how to translate labels and on exactly what behavior we were talking about. The constellation of behaviors that make up CSR has been labeled in a number of different ways since World War I. The only one of these which translated into German, *Kriegsneurose*, or war neurosis, described the more serious forms of breakdown which military psychiatry recognized and treated. The more common forms which today are recognized as comprising CSR had no label and therefore could not be effectively translated into German. Brickenstein stated that if a soldier did break down and could not continue fighting, he was considered a leadership problem, not a problem for medical personnel or psychiatry. In his view, breakdown usually took the form of unwillingness to fight or cowardice.

That the Wehrmacht had good leadership is universally acknowledged. In the early years of the war, without the advantages of numbers of men or material, it accomplished many "impossible" missions. In the later war years, the Wehrmacht defended the country under very unfavorable conditions. For example, in spite of the Russian Army's considerable advantage of men and equipment in the East, Wehrmacht units remained in place and resisted furiously until overwhelmed. Even in seemingly sure defeat, they were able to continue fighting in small groups and slow the Russian advance. This continued far beyond the point at which one would expect total collapse to have occurred.

Only the source of the Wehrmacht's good leadership is disputed. For example, Starry (1983) attributes the excellence of the Wehrmacht to its willingness and ability to change. This ability extended from strategic plans down to small-unit military tactics, making the German Army of World War II one of the finest ever fielded. Although their cause was undoubtedly helped by the Allies' grave strategic blunders, a number of examples show the innovation of the German military; for instance, the adaptation of the tank to ground combat, the fighting doctrine of the *Blitzkrieg*, the rapid march through the "impenetrable" Ardennes in the Meusse Valley, and the use of the Stuka fighter for close combat support.

Wehrmacht leadership has also been discussed in terms of the motivation and tenacity of the individual German soldier, traits that are assumed to be the result of high military cohesion in the small unit. Cohesion, including such things as loyalty, trust, and commitment to peers and leaders enables the small group to sustain itself as a functioning unit even under great stress on the battlefield. Good leaders develop strong military cohesion in a number of ways: they maintain soldiers in small groups which remain together during training and later combat; they show a genuine concern for the soldier's welfare and share in the risks and discomforts of their men; and they ensure that their men are well informed, that is, that there is good communication horizontally and vertically.

Many of the German generals, for example, led their attacks in person. General von Reichenau was the first in his army to cross the Vistula River in the Polish Campaign: he swam it. The Germans were also very effective in building cohesion. Although the Wehrmacht was unquestionably an authoritarian organization, military leaders maintained their positions and at the same time managed to remain close to their subordinates. Shirer (1984) describes the high morale of the Wehrmacht soldier, which

> was based on a camaraderie between officers and men that would have shocked the old Prussian generals and surprised the French, the British, and, I think, the American military of today. . . . For one thing, officers and men were often eating the same food from the same soup kitchen. Officers listened attentively to the reports of enlisted men. The man in charge of the capture of Fort Eban Emeal was a sergeant. When we got to Paris I noticed officers and men off duty sitting at the same table and exchanging talk. In one instance there was a colonel treating a dozen privates to an excellent luncheon. . . . During the repast he discussed with them over a Baedeker the sites of Paris he thought would interest them. Hitler himself, I was also surprised to learn, had drawn up detailed instructions for officers about taking an interest in the personal problems of their men (p 548).

My own interviews of former Wehrmacht noncommissioned officers have confirmed these feelings of camaraderie and the special caring of officers and NCOs for their men. The importance of military cohesion to an effective fighting force was presented some years before World War II in a book entitled *Military Psychology* by Simoneit, a German psychologist (1933). He explained that if a superior was both leader and friend, group cohesion would be much stronger. Furthermore, the leader was responsible for fostering the conviction in each group member that he (the leader) was also a group member. Current German military writing continues to emphasize the importance of the small group to the military (Bundesministerium der Verteidigung, 1980; Poeggeler, 1980) and the integration of new soldiers into the unit (Bastian, 1979; Lippert, Schneider, and Zoll, 1976). These are explicit responsibilities for the small group leader.

Whether the leaders of the Wehrmacht purposely set out to develop strong cohesion is not known, but, they did follow the correct policies for developing it. For example, each division published a booklet detailing the division history and the battle exploits of its individual soldiers. The booklets also included poems and odes to friends and fallen comrades (Die Hammer Division, 1943). A salient theme of these booklets is the importance of comrades. Cohesion is built on shared history, loyalty, and trust of one another. The power of the buddy relations in the Wehrmacht is evident in a book by Lucas (1979) in which he describes the war on the Eastern front from the soldiers' view; "and many, particularly the single men, cut short their leave and returned to those things which were lacking at home: the comradeship of their peers and a sense of purpose." This attitude is especially remarkable in light of the extreme deprivations under which all soldiers fought on the Eastern front.

Other policies that supported the development of strong unit cohesion were the methods of recruitment and replacement. The Wehrmacht recruited soldiers for a division from a single geographic area, thereby capitalizing on prior friendships, acquaintances, customs, and dialects. The recruits were trained together as part of a training battalion by cadre from the division to which they would ultimately be assigned. Such replacements ultimately joined the division as part of a cohesive team. They had had the time to develop loyalty and trust of one another. Because they knew many of their NCOs, as well as division procedures, they probably had a relatively easy time integrating into their new division.

The strong cohesion attributed to Wehrmacht troops presumably greatly reduced the number of combat stress casualties. Today small group cohesion is recognized as one of the most important factors in reducing or preventing stress breakdown. Military cohesion is a multidimensional attribute that includes loyalty, trust, commitment, and psychological support of soldiers for one another, including leaders and subordinates. This protective effect for both military and civilian populations is amply demonstrated in the literature. The exact mechanism through which this effect is mediated is not known, but its efficacy is unquestionable. If small groups in the Wehrmacht were indeed as cohesive as the literature indicates, then low numbers of stress casualties become understandable.

There is yet another explanation for the small number of such casualties, namely, the "good treatment" explanation. Of the few authors who have written about psychiatry during the war, several believe that excellent treatment policies for CSR in the Wehrmacht led to rapid recovery and the prevention of severe cases (Riedesser, 1980). Riedesser, who served in the earlier war, refers to "forward psychiatry" as a development of World War I in which it was found that treating stress casualties close to the front (at what was probably brigade or division clearing stations) led to their rapid return to duty. Thus, "the classic war neuroses did not occur on the German side." As mentioned earlier, forward treatment (proximity) is part of current doctrine for the treatment of CSR. As we will see, it was not again enunciated in the Wehrmacht until fairly late in the war, in spite of Riedesser's recollection.

The good treatment explanation was also provided in a personal interview with another psychiatrist, Von Bayer (1982), who practiced psychiatry in the Sixteenth Army in Russia. He recalled seeing only a few cases of CSR which he assumed were either rapidly cured by good treatment or evacuated and were, therefore, not a serious problem. He recalled discussions and a military psychiatry conference about the CSR problem. Von Bayer pointed out the difficulty of standardizing diagnoses and treatments during the war. He also stated that communication among psychiatrists was very poor and that he never saw the reports or guidelines developed based on the conference he had attended. Curiously, they are available in the German Military Archives.

Valentin (1981) has published a book describing medical problems in the Wehrmacht. In a chapter devoted to psychiatry, he discusses the problem of recognition, labeling, and treatment of behavioral problems, including those that would be called CSR. His data were based on four consecutive annual working congresses for consulting specialists (1941 through 1944). He pointed out that the continuing dilemma of the Wehrmacht physicians was to recognize such cases as psychiatric in origin rather than as organic, and to decide how to label the patients they saw. In those several congresses, no less than four labels for stress reaction were presented, along with a variety of often conflicting diagnoses and treatments. As noted earlier, medical personnel, especially psychiatrists, believed that adverse stress reactions were a leadership rather than a medical problem. This seems to have been the catalyst for a comment on stress in a recent German military guide (Pfister, 1979): "The stress can appear as a breakdown, which *nowadays* we know as an illness and not as cowardice" (p. 12, emphasis added). This was not an area of interest for military psychiatrists; consequently, psychiatrists did not have a shared vocabulary to describe stress symptoms in medical terms or to discuss treatments.

A large number of hysterical trembling cases were seen in World

War I. That trembling, which rendered a soldier unfit for further combat duty, was considered to be a direct outcome of battle stress. But twenty years later medical practice was not prepared to recognize stress reactions, so it is not surprising that physicians had continuing difficulty diagnosing and treating it. Another aspect of this problem has come from Kalinowsky (1950) who interviewed several Wehrmacht psychiatrists immediately after the war. His observations are especially useful because of their timing. He reported that traumatic neuroses (which included what we today call stress reaction) were not considered to be caused by the war experience as such, but by the wish to escape combat and later obtain financial compensation. Years later (1961) Elsaesser also discussed this "secondary gain" (obtaining disability pay). Given the poor communication among physicians and the confused understanding of the cause of the problems they were seeing, even as a rational doctrine for recognition and treatment evolved, its dissemination and application would probably have been stilted. Clearly, stress reactions were not generally believed to be due to human limitations in combat.

Let us now turn to data collected at the German Military Archives. I have selected a representative sample of documents from the years 1939 to 1945 and present them chronologically to demonstrate the Wehrmacht's changing concern about and recognition of CSR. They show the gradual emergence of a treatment policy which is very similar to the one we use today.

On October 19, 1939, the "General Guidance" (*Allgemeine Richtlinien*, 1939) for the duties of military psychiatric consultants was issued. The guidelines included descriptions of the three categories of patients they would likely see: exhaustive neurasthenia, mild psychogenic reaction, and severe psychogenic reaction. The guidelines advised the surgeon general about these patients and also mentioned the *"Kriegsschuettler"* (war trembler), who had been a major problem in World War I. This hysteric reaction to stress manifested itself by uncontrollable shaking which prevented the soldier from further fighting. Psychiatrists were asked to report any occurrences. At about the same time, other guidelines (*Wehrpsychiatrie u. Wehrneurologie*, 1939) were issued which included the statement, "The experiences of the last war make it clear that each of us may react to mental stresses, and if a certain level is reached we no longer are able to withstand them." These documents, therefore, recognized that soldiers could indeed become at least temporarily dysfunctional owing to the stress of battle. But this is the last mention of this possibility found in documents covering at least the next four years. Nazi propaganda probably interceded at this point, and soldier breakdown was not allowed to be discussed in official documents. Most documents discussing behavioral problems in the Wehrmacht were stamped "secret."

Late in 1939, ten military hospitals reported on their experiences with psychiatric patients (Bericht, 1939). One hospital recommended placing soldiers with tremors of hysteric reactions among surgical patients for later transfer to a neuropsychiatric ward. But, at that time, there were few such patients, and they were reported to have had "no real role" in medical practice. At the same time, guidelines were promulgated concerning legal actions for mentally incompetent soldiers (Wuth, 1939). They were first screened to determine whether there was an organic basis for their problems and, if so, to ensure that they were not punished. The screening was also intended to ensure that "psychopaths" (those who did not want to serve, were insubordinate, damaged property, etc.) among them did not get off without punishment. Psychopaths made up a majority of the patients; however, their clinical descriptions closely fit modern descriptions of stress reaction.

Eighteen months later, Elsaesser (1941) referred to "many cases" of "incurable" psychogenic paralysis that he was able to cure by "suggestion" and by administering painful electric shock to the afflicted area. Up to that time he had treated only fourteen patients at his hospital in Ensen. The treatment consisted of suggestion to the soldier that he was not sick and that he could quickly return to duty. The "suggestion" aspect sounds remarkably like our treatment principle of "expectancy," that is, treat the casualty as a soldier who is not sick and who can rapidly return to duty. The electric shock helped speed recovery. A similar treatment, called the Kaufmann technique, was later developed for paralysis of the throat muscles (which prevented the patient from speaking). It is not clear whether this included suggestion or merely painful shock. Ensen soon became a preferred treatment center for soldiers who could not be cured elsewhere.

In late 1941, the collected reports (Wuth, 1941) of sixteen psychiatric consultants (one from each army area) showed that everything was under control. Several mentioned the small number of "hysterics"—the "major problem of the last war"—psychogenics, and psychopaths. It was reported that the "psychiatric measures" seemed to be working. Earlier that year, the same psychiatrists reported on the number of cases of AWOL, desertion, self-mutilation, and self-inflicted wounds they had evaluated for possible legal action. Such cases made up about half the number of patients examined. There was no mention that these problems might relate to stress. If an organic explanation could not be found, imbecility (and consequent sterilization) was a frequent diagnosis. The bases for diagnoses of imbecility were not mentioned. Later in the war, the number and type of these problems increased considerably.

At the end of 1941 the German Army was winnng the war, and so stress casualties assuredly were not considered important and played only a minor medical role. There had been frequent mention of such patients but primarily in the sense of their small number. Treatment consisted of the same kind of care given any other patient and the use of suggestion and shock for the most difficult ones. The cure rate was reported to be quite high, with over 80 percent reportedly returned to duty (Elsaesser, 1961; Van Creveld, 1983). Of these, about two-thirds returned to combat duty. Of special note is the mention of a number of other behaviors (Self-Inflicted Wound, AWOL, suicide) which today would probably be included as manifestations of stress reaction; these problems increased in number in later reports.

In early 1942, a group of psychiatrists reported that the number of war neuroses was not very large, although incidence was slowly increasing (*Beratender Psychiater*, 1943b). No mention was made of how to treat them except for the Ensen shock treatment and the requirement that they be kept out of territorial Germany. This was a propaganda effort to prevent the civilian populace from being negatively affected. Later in that year, "front psychiatry" (treatment of the men near the front) was added as part of the therapy rather than as an adjunct to the propaganda effort. The list of behavioral problems was expanded to include frostbite and venereal disease. Although AWOL, SIW, and insubordination were still considered leadership problems, psychiatrists were required to evaluate them prior to disciplinary action. The interesting additions are frostbite and venereal disease, both of which are preventable but both of which are also far removed from a purely organic basis. Both also belong to the large constellation of behaviors that can comprise CSR.

In April 1942, Bumke wrote that "the number of psychogenic reactions has clearly increased." He was specifically referring to an increase from 1.5 percent to 3.0 percent of patients examined when comparing the last quarter of 1941 with the first quarter of 1942. At that time, there was considerable internal medical correspondence (Kehler, 1942; Pohlisch, 1942a, b; Schneider, 1942; Wuth, 1942a) concerning the first appearance and treatment of the *Schuettel-zitterer* or *Kriegsneurotiker* (trembler and war neurotic, respectively), although the number still seemed to be low. Because of the memories of World War I, they were considered to be a potentially serious problem. The number of hysterical paralysis cases began to increase by that time, and by the middle of 1942 all cases were to be reported directly to Berlin (Schreiber, 1942). Information on the other symptoms mentioned above continued to be reported by psychiatrists. Still, at least one psychiatrist (Richter, 1943) reported that there were fewer psychogenic problems than in World War I. He attributed this to the cohesive attitude of the population, better medical treatment, and education. But he also specifically referred to frostbite and alcohol abuse as self-inflicted wounds. A report for the second quarter of 1942 showed that death sentences for criminal activity had doubled from the previous quarter (Wagner, 1942). Military theft rose 50 percent, AWOL 21 percent, and desertion 53 percent. The possible connection between these behaviors and stress had not been made, and they were still considered a leadership problem.

By September 1942, the Army Chief of Staff became concerned with the problem of soldier attrition. He pointed out that, in 1938, 9.4 percent of discharges were due to nervous or emotional problems, but this figure rose to 18.7 percent in the first six months of 1942 (Handloser, 1942). It is unclear whether this statistic reflected lowered recruitment standards or more frequent and severe reactions on the part of soldiers. Probably both of these variables were in operation, for statistics show markedly different rejection rates among Wehrmacht reception centers. Certainly, recruitment standards must have been lowered, but it is quite possible that the number of reception centers with low rejection rates (presumably leading to recruiting less qualified soldiers) would not have been enough to double the proportion of emotional discharges. These is also considerable evidence that such a recruitment policy is not effective in reducing the number of soldiers who will become stress casualties (Glass, 1973). Therefore, much of the increase was almost certainly due to the greater frequency and severity of stress reactions among the German soldiers.

Evidence for the presence of "war neuroses" became somewhat less equivocal by late 1942. Schneider (1942) referred to the highly contagious nature of psychogenic conditions and the requirement to transfer those who did not respond to treatment to a sanatorium for the duration of the war in order to isolate them. An alternative was to transfer them to special "work battalions" in the occupied zones. This treatment was for those who resisted cure, that is, those who decided it would be better to remain sick than to return to the front. At the same time, the Internal Medical Consultant for Army Group 9 reported, "The psychiatric symptoms reported by Dr. Bansi are less to be blamed on the poor food than on the effects of various stress factors (constant terror, little sleep, living in dirty and wet conditions)" (p. 2). In addition, the report comments on the large number of soldiers who had trouble controlling their bowels and bladder (*Beratender Psychiater*, 1943a). This is the first direct reference, since 1939, to the role of stress in generating behavioral problems among combat soldiers.

Finally, in March 1943, the surgeon general (Handloser, 1943) reported: "We have discovered that the number of psychogenic disturbances is increasing as the war goes on." This marked the beginning of greatly increased concern in this area. Late in 1942, Dr. Panse, who worked at the Ensen hospital, was asked to make a film on war hysterics. It was to show how psychogenics, in this case those with hysteric conversion reactions, could be successfully cured using the suggestion/shock treatment, and how easy it was to mistake psychogenic reactions for organic injury (Christukat, 1943b; Panse, 1942; Wuth, 1942b). The film was made to help educate general medical officers on soldiers' psychogenic reactions in combat. Recognition and treatment were to be emphasized. At last, military physicians were to have some help in responding to a problem that was only then beginning to be officially recognized.

At about this time, the office of the surgeon general emphasized the need to keep "war neurotics" from being transported to the rear. (*Der Heeres-Sanitaetsinspekteur Heeresarzt*, 1943). Although this policy is similar to the application of the principle of proximity, it was motivated by a belief that such cases would be a poor influence on morale. But a more telling part of the report shows the added concern about the number of stress casualties in an army with diminishing resources: "Also, the timely recognition, correct treatment, and use of soldiers with nervous/mental disturbances is—at least in this fourth year of the war—moving into importance" (p. 1). By early that year, field experience with rising numbers of stress casualties must have become quite common.

Other psychiatrists reported on their experiences in recognizing and treating stress casualties. In a hand-dated document (*Psychiatrie und Neurologie*, 1943), an unidentified military psychiatrist wrote a paper describing treatment for CSR. The first step in the therapy was to get help from the physician and his buddies. If that didn't work, the patient was to be transferred to a hospital or the rear lines for a minimum of eight days where he received food and rest. Sleep-inducing drugs were also administered. After eight days, the psychiatrist wrote, the soldier should be able to be returned to duty. "Buddy aid" (*Kameradschaftliche Zusprache*) and the supportive behavior of personnel around the casualty were important factors in treatment. Although current treatment doctrine does not include early evacuation, it, too, emphasizes the importance of buddy aid and rest and the expectation of fairly early return to duty. These were officially recognized in July 1943 (Wuth, 1943) in guidelines released from Berlin. They emphasized the importance of immediate treatment (immediacy), rest, and "buddy aid" (simplicity) at the front (proximity) as part of the treatment.

Also in the middle of 1943, the script for the film about psychogenic casualties was completed. The film refers to the error of looking for an organic basis for hysteric disturbances during World War I and to the problems the French had had with psychogenic stomach cramps. For the first time, reference was made to psychogenic battle reactions as "normal":

Now, at the front, psychogenic reactions are treated objectively and caught in time so that, in almost all cases, hysteric reactions can be avoided. Most were sent back to their units: one realizes that a one-time collapse during the "baptism of fire" is usually neither hysteria nor can it be thought of as cowardice (Panse, 1943, p. 3).

This represented a remarkable change in the official attitude toward breakdown in battle. By 1943 all aspects of current treatment doctrine for stress casualties had been stated. Most had been officially recognized by Berlin, but they were apparently not well disseminated among treatment personnel and so there remained disbelievers. A military psychiatric consultant in Paris still reported that hysteric reactions were not a problem and made up about two cases per thousand men during the third quarter of that year (Rhode, 1943). He made no mention of other labels and diagnoses that had by then been recognized. Malingering was added to the list of psychogenic reactions monitored by psychiatrists.

The general picture concerning combat stress had cleared by the end of 1943. The concepts of immediate treatment, forward treatment, early return to duty, and "buddy aid" had appeared. In addition, stress reaction as a "normal" consequence of battle was recognized. Several recent German military reports on coping with stress in combat specifically mention the role of fear (Pfister, 1979). But late in 1943, stress reaction was only beginning to be doctrinally recognized. Recognition, treatment, definitions, and labels continued to be a problem. Wehrmacht psychiatrists continued to suffer from inadequate sharing of information on this topic. However, a report from one military hospital (Ensen) demonstrated increased proportions of patients admitted due to psychological stress problems (Figure 4.1). "Psychopathic and hysterical" diagnoses made up 25 percent of admissions by the end of 1943. (Only diagnoses not related to injury or disease appear in this table. These data are not representative of all hospitals, for Ensen had become a preferred center for treating CSR casualties.) Other evidence for the increased recognition of this problem came from the surgeon general who in 1944 released a report on troop hospitalizations (Handloser, 1944). It listed the twelve most important categories of illness for 1942 and 1935. In 1942 "mental illness," which included many of the same symptoms which we today call CSR, was ranked sixth out of twelve, accounting for 6 percent of all admissions. This percentage was six times greater than it was in 1935, when it was ranked eleventh out of twelve as a cause of hospitalization.

In March of 1944 the psychiatric consultant for Munich forwarded a document (Grosse, 1944) to the surgeon general which was to be used for instruction to the officer corps concerning the *Kriegszitterer* (war trembler). Shortly thereafter, another psychiatric consultant (Bumke, 1944) reported: "The number of war neurotics has risen to such a large amount within the last months that I find it important to report solely on this condition" (p. 1). He presented figures demonstrating that the number had doubled, although denominators were not given. He also wrote: "One must add to these numbers those hysterics who

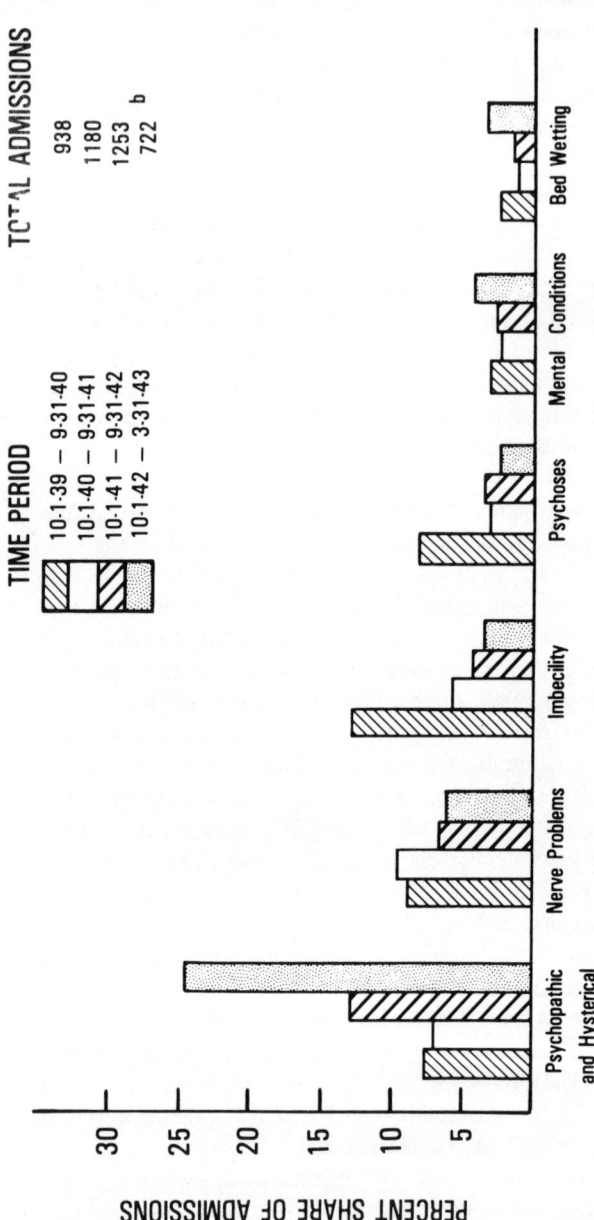

Figure 4.1
Diagnoses of Patients Admitted to the Ensen Military Hospital[a]

are in the occupied territories and in Army hospitals as well as those who are patients in other hospitals but unrecognized as such" (p. 1). This is an important point for two reasons. First, it demonstrates a clear understanding of the extent of the problem and, second, it demonstrates an understanding of the difficulty of its recognition. Following his argument, one could add the numbers who were treated as hospital outpatients and the number who were treated at the unit level through buddy aid or the local physician. Dr. Bumke made a strong plea that such patients be treated as ambulatory patients and not as if they were ill. This was an unambiguous statement of the expectancy principle. He went on to describe bed wetting, vomiting, and gastrointestinal problems as "psychogenic, stress related problems." Gastrointestinal problems and certain headaches were added to the list of problems psychiatrists were to monitor.

Following Bumke's report, the Office of the Surgeon General (1944) requested a separate report on the number of soldiers with psychogenic disturbances. At the same time, Panse, a psychiatric consultant, reported a "tripling of psychogenics after the invasion, although the numbers are still small, namely, one out of 10,000 soldiers" (Panse, 1944a). His rates were considerably lower (only one tenth as large) than those reported from the Western front six months earlier. Panse continually reported that the number of psychogenic reactions was not large. In March 1944, however, he acknowledged that psychogenic problems had become more frequent in the field army outside of Germany (Panse, 1944b) in contrast to the relatively combat-free interior of Germany (Barvaria) where he worked.

Evidence for the seriousness of the problem was becoming hard to ignore or deny by the middle of 1944. Apparently, a kind of evacuation syndrome (Belenky and Jones, 1981) began to emerge, as it offered an honorable way out of the war. An information sheet for line officers (*Anlage IV*, 1944) stated: "Unnecessarily, and in dangerous amounts, cases are multiplying where officers and soldiers are delaying their recoveries from illnesses, wounds, and accidents for a long period of time. . . . These people were known as 'war hysterics' even as far back as the first war." (I found no other earlier references to this type of war hysteric in any other document.) But the trial-and-error learning of an effective treatment doctrine was by that time almost complete. The Office of the Surgeon General soon released another statement (Wuth, 1944) concerning treatment for stress reaction which is almost identical to present-day doctrine: "The treatment of such disturbances is at first in the unit, right after the start of the hysteric reaction, using quiet but determined comradely comfort (buddy aid) and rest periods of short duration." This demonstrates the principles of proximity (treat the casualty close to the front), simplicity (buddy aid), expectancy (the soldier will return to duty after a brief rest), and immediacy (treat the casualty right away). This official paper from the surgeon general was probably issued too late to have much impact. Communication problems further restricted its dissemination.

An increasing proportion of psychiatric reports were devoted to the problem of combat reaction throughout 1944. Although a few reports continued to deemphasize the problem, the large majority acknowledged it. Many suggested treatment alternatives. During that year, the concept of ambulatory treatment was introduced, and the principles of proximity, expectancy, immediacy, and simplicity were clearly enunciated. The full range of medical behaviors which today are included as stress-related were included in the Wehrmacht list of "psychogenic" disturbances. Nonetheless, the appropriate treatment for stress reaction was still being debated in early 1945. The difficulty of communication impeded further progress in establishing a treatment doctrine. One consultant suggested that esprit de corps was important in preventing and treating psychiatric disturbance (DeCrinis, 1945). This was the first time that a psychiatrist stated the connection between a corollary of cohesion (esprit de corps) and the problem of stress reactions.

The process of learning to recognize and treat the combat stress casualty proceeded slowly in the Wehrmacht. The first step in this process was recognition. The Wehrmacht psychiatrist failed on this account because of his lack of training, a lack that may be attributed to the influence of the organic psychiatry movement which emphasized the wrong causes for combat breakdown, as well as to political influences which affected how he viewed behavior and leadership. The number of stress casualties eventually became overwhelming, and recognition of the magnitude of the problem seems to have been widespread. But then came the problem of developing an efficacious treatment doctrine. Although this development did occur, it was not widely disseminated, having been "discovered" bit by bit by a number of psychiatrists practicing in the combat zones in a losing war effort. The war gradually became closer, and, as strategic communications were disrupted, nonessential communication surely suffered even more. Thus, a centrally recognized and disseminated doctrine did not occur until late 1944. The problems of recognition were further exacerbated by two other beliefs: (1) good leadership could prevent the kind of stress reaction that had been seen in World War I, and (2) high-quality medical intervention could rapidly cure any behavioral problems that emerged. Because both military leadership and medical practice were assumed to be good, stress breakdown, or war neurosis, was neither expected nor planned for.

We have few good statistics to demonstrate actual rates of stress breakdown in the German Army. For the most part, the numbers that are available do not have denominators, so rates cannot be calculated. Some readers might challenge these conclusions, on the basis that I have not included many such rates. Yet a large group of military psychiatrists (and others involved in personnel areas) from throughout the Wehrmacht reported that the number of stress casualties was increasing as the war went on. In all probability, the actual size of the German Army was decreasing as casualties outnumbered accessions. This would mean that overall rates must have been increasing. Furthermore, it is unreasonable to expect "hard" statistics for a medical problem that was neither defined nor anticipated. It is only through the continued reports of a number of medical practitioners that such a problem can be discovered. By the end of the war, it was more than merely "discovered": it was a pervasive topic of reports, meetings, and official guidelines. Unfortunately, Panse (1944a), who continually downplayed the role of stress breakdown in the Wehrmacht, is one of the few psychiatrists who did report denominators. His widely quoted statistic of one case per ten thousand soldiers was based on his experience in Bavaria, one of the few areas of Germany that escaped heavy fighting. This statistic seems to contradict his own efforts to produce a film documenting the "acceptable" breakdown of soldiers during their first combat experience.

CONCLUSION

The widespread perception that the Wehrmacht did not suffer serious problems of soldier breakdown owing to battle stress can be successfully challenged. The Germans were not specifically interested in preventing combat stress reaction; however, there can be little doubt that they did what we would now recognize as optimal. They built well-integrated units that almost certainly had the high level of cohesion necessary to reduce the impact of battle stress on the soldier. But in spite of good leadership, in spite of the refusal to accept the idea of combat stress reaction, and in spite of some fairly harsh treatment for what was indeed stress reaction, stress casualties developed into a serious and pervasive problem.

REFERENCES

Albee, G. W. (1985). The answer is prevention. *Psychology Today*, February, 60–62.
Allgemeine Richtlinien fuer die Taetigkeit des Beratenden Psychiaters. (1939). Berlin, October 19, Militaerarchiv, Freiburg.
Anlage IV, Merkblatt fuer die Truppenoffiziere. (c, 1944). Militaerarchiv, Freiburg.
Bar-on, R., Soloman, Z., Noy, S., and Nardi, C. (1983). *War related stress: an overview of the clinical picture in the 1982 conflict in Lebanon*. Paper presented at the Third International Conference on Psychological Stress and Adjustment in Time of War and Peace, Tel Aviv, Israel, January 4.
Bastian, H. D. (1979). Militaerische Menchenfuehrung in Kleinen Gruppen. *Kontakte*, Ausbildungshilfe der Schule der Bundeswehr fuer Innere Fuehrung, BMVg.
Beebe, G. W., and Appel, J. W (1958). *Variation is psychological tolerance to ground combat in World War II*. Washington, D.C.: Medical Research and Development Branch, Office of the Surgeon General, Department of the Army.
Belenky, G. L., and Jones, F. D. (1981). Evacuation syndromes in military exercises: a model of the psychiatric casualties of combat. In *Proceedings, Users Workshop on Combat Stress*. Fort Sam Houston, Tex.: Academy of Health Sciences, September 2-4, 140–142.
Belenky, G. L., Jones, F. D., and Newhouse, P. (1981). *Military psychiatry in future wars*. Paper presented at the meeting of the American Psychiatric Association, New Orleans, La.
Belenky, G. L., Noy, S., and Soloman, Z. (1985). Battle stress: the Israeli experience. *Military Review*, 65, 29–37.
Beratender Psychiater beim Heeres-Sanitaetsinspekteur (Consulting Psychiatrist, OTSG). (1943a). "Bericht-d. Ber. Internisten beim Armeearzt 9 v. 30.12.42 ueber das vorkommen von Erschoepfungen," Berlin, April 14, Militaerarchiv, Freiburg.

MILITARY PSYCHIATRY IN THE GERMAN ARMY 143

Beratender Psychiater beim Heeres-Sanitaetsinspekteur (Consulting Psychiatrist, OTSG). (1943b). "Sammelbericht 2," Berlin, February, Militaerarchiv, Freiburg.

"Bericht" (of army hospitals at Baumholder, Wiesbaden, Kiedrich, Mainz, Darmstadt, Jugenheim, and field hospitals at Birkenfeld, St. Wendel, Heidelberg, and Wieblingen). (1939). November 12, Militaerarchiv, Freiburg.

Brickenstein, R. Personal interview (E. O'Brien). (1982). Freiburg, February.

Bumke to the Surgeon General. (1942). Subject: "Berichterstattung der Beratenden Aerzte," Munich, April 1, Militaerarchiv, Freiburg.

Bumke to the Surgeon General. (1944). Subject: "Berichterstattung der Beratenden Aerzte," Munich, April 4, Militaerarchiv, Freiburg.

Bundesministerium der Verteidigung. (1980). *Die Ersten Stunden*. Hinweise fuer die Vorgesetzten. Schriftenreihe innere Fuehrung BMVg, *Heft 9*.

Christukat to Dr. Panse. (1943a). Subject: "Filmaufnahmen von psychogenen Bewegungsstoerungen," Berlin, January 20, Militaerarchiv, Freiburg.

Christukat to Dr. Wuth. (1943b). No subject line, Berlin, April 30, Militaerarchiv, Freiburg.

Cocks, G. (1985). *Psychotherapy in the Third Reich*. New York: Oxford University Press.

DeCrinis, M. to Reichsarzt SS. (1945). No subject line, Berlin, February 9; with enclosure "Stellungnahme zur Anweisung fuer Truppenaerzte ueber 'Erkennung und Behandlung von abnormen seelischen Reaktionen (Neurose)' von OFA Prof. Dr. J. H. Schultz." Berlin, February 8, Militaerarchiv, Freiburg.

Der Heeres-Sanitaetsinspekteur Heeresarzt (Schmidt, Oberfeldarzt). (1943). "Verfuegungs-Entwurf," April 9, Militaerarchiv, Freiburg.

Die Hammer Division, Suedlich des Ilmensee. (1943). Rigaer Druckerei, December.

Elsaesser, G. (1941). "Bericht des Ass.-Arztes: Dr. Elsaesser ueber Heilungen von hysterischen Laehmungen and Reaktionen durch hohe galvanische Stroeme (unter Anwendung von Suggestivmassnahmen)," Ensen, July 7, Militaerarchiv, Freiburg.

Elsaesser, G. (1961). "Erfahrung an 1400 Kriegsneurosen." *Psychiatrie der Gegenwart*, Springer Verlag, *III*, 623–630.

Glass, A. J. (1954). Psychotherapy in the combat zone. *American Journal of Psychiatry*, *110*, 725–731.

Glass, A. J. (1955). Principles of combat psychiatry. *Military Medicine*, *117*, 27–33.

Glass, A. J. (1973). Lessons learned. In W. S. Mullens and A. J. Glass (eds.), *Neuropsychiatry in World War II: Vol. 2. Overseas theaters*. Washington, D.C.: U.S. Government Printing Office, 989–1027.

Grosse to the Surgeon General. (1944). Subject: "Behandlung der Kriegszitterer," Munich, March 18, Militaerarchiv, Freiburg.
Handloser to Wehrkreis commanders I-XIII, XX, and XXI. (1942). No subject line, Berlin, September 26, Militaerarchiv, Freiburg.
Handloser to corps surgeons. (1943). Subject: "Behandlung von Soldaten mit hysterischen und psychogenen Reaktionen," Berlin, February 9, Militaerarchiv, Freiburg.
Handloser. (1944). *Der Heeres-Sanitaetsinspekteur*, Nr. 1249/44 geh. (Wi G Ib). Berlin, January 30, Militaerarchiv, Freiburg.
Ingraham, L. H., and Manning, F. J. (1980). Psychiatric battle casualties: The missing column in a war without replacements. *Military Review*, August 19-29.
Kalinowsky, L. B. (1950). War and post-war neuroses in Germany. *Medical Bulletin of the U.S. Army, Europe*, March, 7, No. 3.
Kehrer to Dr. Wuth. (1942). No subject line, Muenster, April 1, Militaerarchiv, Freiburg.
Lippert, E., Schneider, P., and Zoll, R. (1976). Sozialisation in der Bundeswehr: Der Einfluss des Wehrdienstes auf soziale und politische Einstellungen der Wehrpflichtigen. *Schriftenreihe Innere Fuehrung*, BMVg, Heft 25.
Lucas, J. (1979). *War on the Eastern Front, 1941-1945: The German soldier in Russia*. Briarcliff Manor, N.Y.: Stein & Day.
Madej, W. V. (1978). Effectiveness and cohesion of the German ground forces in World War II. *Journal of Political and Military Sociology*, 6, 233–249.
Noy, S. (1982). Division based psychiatry in intensive war situations. *Journal of the Royal Army Medical Corps*, 128, 105–116.
Office of the Surgeon General. (1944). To all corps and Wehrkreis surgeons, Subject: 'Meldungen ueber psychogene Stoerungen," Berlin, July 3, 1944, Militaerarchiv, Freiburg.
Panse to Dr. Wuth. (1942). Subject: "nr. 4362/42," Ensen (Cologne), December 28, 1942, Militaerarchiv, Freiburg.
Panse to Dr. Wuth. (1943). Cover letter to film script: Ensen, November 20, Militaerarchiv, Freiburg.
Panse. (1944a). "Durchschrift des Tagebuchs des Beratenden San.-Offiziers, Ensen, October 4, Militaerarchiv, Freiburg.
Panse. (1944b). "Auszugsweise Abschrift aus dem Bericht des Beratenden Psychiaters beim Wehrkreis VI Reserve-Lazarett Ensen bei Koeln, den 12 Januar 1944," March 15, Militaerarchiv, Freiburg.
Pfister, U. (1979). Psychisches Versagen im Kampf. *Allg Schweiz Mil*, May, 145–145, 249–253.
Poeggeler, F. (1980). Menchenfuehrung in der Bundeswehr. Ausbildung der

Vorgesetzten in der Bundeswehr auf dem Gebiet der Menchenfuehrung. *Schriftenreihe innere Feuhrung*, BMVg, Heft 1.
Pohlisch to Dr. Wuth. (1942a). Subject: "Schuttel-Zitterer oder Kriegsneurotiker," Bonn. April 4, Militaerarchiv, Freiburg.
Pohlisch to Dr. Wuth. (1942b). No subject line, Bonn, April 17, Militaerarchiv, Freiburg.
"Psychiatrie und Neurologie." (1943). Hand-dated February 15, Militaerarchiv, Freiburg (document number H 20 1488).
Richter to Berichtsammelstelle der Militaeraerztlichen Akademie, Berlin. (1943). Subject: "Erfahrungsbericht des Beratenden Psychiaters," May 12, Militaerarchiv, Freiburg.
Riedesser, P. (1980). Militaerpsychiatrie und psychologie. *Handwoerterbuch der Psychologie*, Weinheim, FRG: Beltz.
Rock, S. K., and Schneider, R. J. (1984). Battle stress reactions and the Israeli experience in Lebanon: a brief summary. *Medical Bulletin of the U.S. Army, Europe*, 41(1), 9–11.
Rohde. (1943). "Vierteljaehrlicher Erfahrungsbericht fuer die Zeit vom 1.10-31.12.43," Paris, January 10, Militaerarchiv, Freiburg.
Schneider, C. (1942). "Bericht des Beratenden Psychiaters im Wehrkreis XII," Heidelberg, October 21, Militaerarchiv, Freiburg.
Schneider, R. J., and Luscomb, R. L. (1984). Battle stress reaction and the United States Army. *Military Medicine*, 149, 66–69.
Schreiber to Wehrkreis physicians I-XIII, XVII, XX, XXI. (1942). Subject: "Meldung von Kriegszitterern an Beratende Psychiater beim Ersatzheer." (1942). Berlin, July 31, Militaerarchiv, Freiburg.
Shirer, W. L. (1984). *The nightmare years*. Boston: Little, Brown.
Simoneit, M. (1933). *Wehrpsychologie*. Berlin: Bernard & Graeffe.
Starry, D. A. (1983). To change an army. *Military Review*, March, 20–27.
Valentin, R. (1981). *Die Krankenbattallione*. Dusseldorf, FRG: Droste.
Van Creveld, M. (1983). *Fighting power: German and U.S. Army performance 1939–1945*. Westport, Conn.: Greenwood Press.
Von Bayer, (1982). Personal interview (E. O'Brien), Ueberlingen-Bodensee, June.
Wagner to Wuth. (1942). Subject: "Kriegs-Kriminalstatistik," Berlin, August, 20, Militaerarchiv, Freiburg.
"Wehrpsychiatrie und Wehrpsychologie." (1939). October 10, Militaerarchiv, Freiburg.
Wuth, O. (1939). 'Denkschrift betreffend die Zubilligung des Paragraph 51 RStGB, Absatz 1 und 2 seitens der fachaerztlich psychiatrisch ausgebildeten Sanitaetsoffiziere sowie betreffend die aus der Zubilligung des Paragraph 51 Absatz 1 und 2 zu ziehenden Folgerungen," probably, Militaerarchiv, Freiburg.

Wuth, O. (1941). "Sammelbericht des Beratenden Psychiaters beim Heers-Sanitaetsinspekteur," Berlin, November 4, Militaerarchiv, Freiburg.
Wuth, O. to Dr. Panse. (1942). No subject line, Berlin, December 9, Militaerarchiv, Freiburg.
Wuth, O. (1943). "Richtlinien fuer die Beurteilung von Soldaten mit seelischnervoesen Abartigkeiten ('Psychopathen') und seelischnervoesen Reaktionen sowie fuer die Ueberweisung in Sonderabteilungen," July 21, Militaerarchiv, Freiburg.
Wuth, O. (c. 1944). "Voraussetzungen zur Behandlung von Soldaten mit reaktiven hysterischen Stoerungen," Berlin, Militaerarchiv, Freiburg.

5

Military Psychiatry in the Israeli Defense Force

GREGORY LUCAS BELENKY

Psychiatric casualties are a large source of manpower loss in modern warfare. They were first well described in the beginning of this century. Since then, much has been learned about the nature, prevention, and treatment of psychiatric casualties from anecdotal accounts, from trial-and-error clinical treatment, and from both retrospective and prospective studies. The formula of prevention based on good morale, treatment based on immediate attention near the front, and rapid return to combat duty is a useful distillation of the experiences of the past. This may suggest, incorrectly, that everything needed is known about the nature, prevention, and treatment of combat psychiatric casualties. As conflicts become shorter, more intense, and more fluid, however, psychiatric casualties emerge more rapidly, appearing within hours after the beginning of hostilities. Treating pscyhiatric casualties near the front and returning them to duty become more difficult. The importance of combat psychiatry, while remembered in principle, tends to be forgotten in the practical business of planning for possible future wars.

The experiences of the Israelis during the 1973 Arab-Israeli War

The views of the author do not purport to reflect the positions of the department of the army or the department of defense (Para 4-3, AR-360-5).

and the 1982 war in Lebanon have confirmed the basic principles of combat psychiatry. In addition, new information has emerged which refines these principles and suggests important, unanswered questions on the nature, treatment, and prevention of combat psychiatric casualties.

BATTLE-SHOCK IN THE 1973 ARAB-ISRAELI WAR

The 1973 Arab-Israeli War was short and intense. It lasted approximately four weeks, caused heavy casualties, consumed vast quantities of military materiel, and in its early phases was fought twenty-four hours a day. Battles were mobile and fluid, with armor, infantry, artillery, and air support attempting to work in close coordination. The Israelis were taken by surprise, nearly overrun by sheer numbers of men and masses of equipment, and initially forced to retreat. Even as they were retreating, the Israelis fought resourcefully and tenaciously with great tactical flexibility and personal initiative. Owing in part to the inflexibility of their adversaries, the Israelis were able to mobilize their reserves, gain tactical initiative, and exploit it to regain their original positions.

The Israeli Defense Force (IDF) suffered a relatively high rate of psychiatric casualties (termed "battle-shock" casualties in this chapter) during the 1973 war. Psychiatric casualties in battle are generally expressed as a ratio of the psychiatric casualties to the wounded in action. Immediately after the war, the ratio of psychiatric casualties to wounded in action (WIA) was given officially as 14:100 or 12.5 percent of all nonfatal casualties. Upon reexamination, however, the Israelis found this figure to be low: the actual ratio was approximately 30:100, or 23 percent of all nonfatal casualties. The revised figure includes those formally recorded as battle-shock (the originally reported 12.5 percent of casualties), those not formally so recorded but nevertheless suffering from battle-shock, some late reactions, and battle-shock in the wounded.

The 1973 war was the first in which the Israelis sustained significant numbers of battle-shock casualties. In prior wars, the number of such casualties had been low, treatment informal, and hence, at the time of the 1973 war, no formal doctrinal or organizational provisions were made for the treatment of battle-shock. As a result, during the 1973 war, all battle-shock casualties were evacuated to the rear. Most were treated in civilian hospitals, and only a few returned to combat duty during the war. For many, recovery was slow and disability prolonged.

The Israelis were stunned by the suddenness and intensity of the attack and by the number of physical and psychiatric casualties sustained in the 1973 war. The conflict was described by the IDF surgeon general as a demographic disaster for Israel, because so many capable people were killed. The rate of battle-shock casualties was high relative to their experience in prior wars. Following the war, in cooperation with Israeli academic institutions, the IDF subjected itself to intense scrutiny. It was hampered by a lack of systematic recordkeeping during the war, as a result of which valuable information was lost. Nevertheless, the results of this self-scrutiny led to the development of doctrine for treating battle-shock casualties and for collecting better combat data. These were subsequently applied during the 1982 war in Lebanon.

The Israelis reviewed the literature on combat psychiatry and combined their own observations from the war with those of others from previous wars into a coherent clinical picture of combat psychiatric casualties (Noy, 1978a). They drew a distinction between battle-shock ("combat reaction" in Israeli terminology) and battle fatigue. Battle-shock, defined as a simple emotional reaction to the stress of battle, developed after hours or days of intense combat. In contrast, battle fatigue developed after weeks or months of moderate combat. In the 1973 war and later in the 1982 war in Lebanon, psychiatric casualties took the form of battle-shock. Battle-shock progressed through three stages. The first or immediate stage lasted hours to days and was characterized by anxiety, depression, and fear. The majority of soldiers with battle-shock recovered during the immediate stage. Those who did not recover passed into the second, or acute stage, which was characterized by the emergence of neurotic symptoms consistent with the soldier's prewar personality. This stage lasted for days to weeks and recovery was still likely. If treatment in the acute stage failed, the soldier passed into the third, or chronic stage which was characterized by personality impoverishment and chronic psychiatric disability. This stage was of extended duration and recovery was slow and often incomplete.

In the 1973 war, a new form of battle psychiatric casualty emerged: delayed battle-shock. Some soldiers who had done well during intense fighting broke down upon receiving their first telephone call from home, or broke down when home on their first leave. Delayed battle-shock also emerged in another form. This other form occurred on the Suez front. Battle-shock casualties on this front were evacuated to military hospitals in the middle of the Sinai. There, soldiers suffering battle-shock rested for twenty-three days, recovered, and were ready to return to duty. However, because no provision had been made to return them to their units, the men were then evacuated to Tel Aviv or Jerusalem. These soldiers frequently suffered second, more serious, decompensations during the latter evacuation.

The Israelis observed that the intensity of fighting, more so than its duration, produced battle-shock. Battle-shock cases were numerous during the first hours and days of the 1973 war, and highest during the crossing of the Suez Canal when indirect fire (artillery and rockets) was the most intense. When intensity was extreme, battle-shock emerged in the first few hours of fighting, before the onset of significant fatigue or sleep deprivation. Parenthetically, even under the most severe battle conditions, Israeli soldiers appeared to manage three to four hours of sleep in every twenty-four. The risk of battle-shock, in addition to varying with battle intensity, varied, in combat units, with the soldier's combat role. Battle-shock was most prevalent in armored units, intermediately prevalent in artillery units, and least prevalent in infantry units. The high prevalence in armored units was probably a result of their being engaged in the most intense combat. Reservists were more vulnerable than active service soldiers. Soldiers from support units were more vulnerable than combat troops. Thus, battle intensity, primarily, and the soldier's battle role, secondarily, were the factors related to battle-shock.

The Israelis conducted a retrospective examination of forty IDF soldiers who suffered battle-shock during the 1973 war (Noy, 1978b). Each had received treatment during the acute stage of the syndrome. With regard to completeness of recovery, as of a year or two after the war, 45 percent had no difficulties, 31 percent had some difficulties, 21 percent had many difficulties, and 3 percent had severe difficulties. Thirty-five percent of the men with battle-shock had been seriously wounded. In 70 percent of this wounded group, the physical injury was a direct cause of the battle-shock. Forty percent of the men with battle-shock reported having interpersonal difficulties in their units, contrasted with 10 percent in a control group of men not suffering battle-shock. Prior or ongoing civil stresses were found in 80 percent of the cases of battle-shock. Fifty percent of the cases had wives who were pregnant or who had given birth within the year preceding the war. In 23 percent of the cases, there had been a recent death in the immediate family. Other apparently relevant civil stresses were being newly married, taking on a mortgage, having sick parents, or undergoing a serious personal loss. Neither the presence nor the severity of either combat or civilian stresses bore any relationship to likelihood of recovery from the immediate or the acute stage.

There was, however, a significant correlation between the soldier's normal personality and prognosis. For the purposes of the study, a soldier was classified as having a stable, a transitional, or a repressed personality. Well-adjusted men in untroubled life circumstance were classified as stable. Men facing developmental crises, generally in their late teens or late thirties and early forties, were classified as transitional. Men who dealt with anger or anxiety with repression, and denied having felt anger at any time in their adult lives (self-reports confirmed through interviews with their families), were classified as emotionally repressed. As civilians, those with repressed personalities lived in communities containing large numbers of transient persons, communities in which there was significant personal and group maladjustment. Those soldiers with repressed personalities had the poorest prognosis for recovery among the three types; those with transitional personalities had a somewhat better prognosis; and those with stable personalities had the best prognosis and generally recovered from the acute stage (Noy, 1978b).

The above study concluded that prior or ongoing civil stresses modulated the potency of battle stresses in generating battle-shock. Soldiers who had stressful home situations, for reasons ranging from recent births to recent deaths, were more vulnerable to battle-shock. Personality type was not a predictor of becoming a psychiatric casualty. Once breakdown occurred, however, soldiers with better adjusted personalities were more likely to recover.

The Israelis also did a retrospective comparison of social supports, both military and civilian, between soldiers who suffered battle-shock and those who emerged from intense battle psychiatrically unscathed (Steiner and Neumann, 1978). In contrast to the unscathed group, the men who suffered battle-shock reported little or no identification with their unit or team, no trust in their leadership, frequent transfer and rotation, feelings of loneliness and of not belonging to their unit, and finally, low self-esteem regarding their military performance. It appeared that all of the above factors contributed to the development of battle-shock. In contrast, positive social support, group identification, stability of assignment, and high regard for one's work appeared to protect against battle-shock even during intense fighting.

The Israelis found two treatments for battle-shock described in the combat psychiatry literature. One consisted of rest and supportive psychotherapy at or near the front and a rapid return to combat duty. Supportive psychotherapy entails a brief recounting of events by the patient, coupled with reassurance from the therapist. The second treatment consisted of releasing tension and suppressed emotions through extensive conscious examination and by reliving the combat trauma in imagination, words, or abreaction. In psychoanalytic terms, this latter treatment is called abreaction. The method of a brief rest and return to duty has been used near the front in military medical units. The method of abreaction has been used in rear areas in civilian hospitals. Until the Israeli review, no attempt had been made to integrate these two techniques and to provide differential indications for their use (Noy, 1978a). The review suggested that rest and support near the front, and abreaction in the rear, were appropriate therapy for different stages of battle-shock. Accordingly, rest and supportive psychotherapy with rapid return to combat duty is the treatment of choice for the immediate stage of battle-shock, but if this treatment fails and the person passes into the acute stage, then evacuation to the rear and abreaction are indicated.

Most 1973 battle-shock casualties, whether they broke down at the front, on the way home, or at home, were treated in civilian hospitals. Treatment in a civilian hospital clearly promoted disability: soldiers on the verge of coping were undermined by the acceptance, pity, and empathy of the civilian hospital staff. These observations underscored the value of prompt, brief treatment near the front and rapid return to duty.

The Israelis analyzed the situational and personal variables associated with heroic behavior (Gal, 1978). They found no personality type prone to heroism; rather, they found that certain situations invariably called forth heroic behavior. Aspects of these hero-producing situations were good leadership, strong unit cohesion, and intense combat stress. They studied seventy-two soldiers who received medals for valor during the 1973 Arab-Israeli War. These soldiers were compared to a control group matched by unit and rank on a variety of measures of personality, performance, and cognitive ability. In turn, each heroic act was studied for the presence or absence of a number of variables: isolation, being in command, commander present, saving the wounded, type of battle, heroic act as the result of an explicit command, being surrounded, few against many, and saving the lives of others.

Analysis of the personal characteristics of the medal recipients revealed that age most readily distinguished the heroes from the nonheroes: the heroes were younger. Associated findings were that the heroes were less often married and, if married, less likely to have children. The heroes also showed higher intelligence, motivation, overall rating on personality factors, and higher army course scores. There were no differences in educational achievement or physical fitness.

The situational factors associated with heroic acts were analyzed statistically. Four clusters of situational variables were associated with heroic acts: in the first cluster, the men were surrounded, outnumbered, defending, and retreating. They were acting together when the heroic act was performed. The commander was the hero, or the commander was present; the heroic act occurred while breaking out of an encirclement. In the second cluster, the men were in a face-to-face battle and the hero was saving the lives of the wounded. The commander was absent and the hero was psychologically isolated from his comrades. The hero remained alive while saving others. In the third cluster, the men were a few against the many. It was the hero's regular unit, and he died saving the lives of his friends. The fourth cluster found the hero alone, fighting in an offensive battle to the last bullet. He was not under clear orders. He was not fighting to save himself or others. He died alone. Ten to twenty cases fit into each cluster. The clusters accounted for approximately two-thirds of the cases of heroism. The remaining cases were sufficiently unique that common situational factors did not emerge.

The Israelis concluded that heroes were not clearly distinguishable from nonheroes. They fell generally into the upper quartile of overall scores and test results. The heroes were generally officers or noncommissioned officers who had good, but not perfect, military records. Most had shown some resistance to military authority in the form of being absent without leave, or being disciplined for breaches of military regulations at some point in their military service. The Israelis concluded that there was no specific personality associated with being a medal recipient, and that with regard to personality "we all are at risk for heroism" (Gal, 1978).

The results of the above study show that heroes are not unique and that certain characteristic situations call forth heroism. In all of these situations, the heroes were involved in intense combat. In the first three of the four situational clusters, and perhaps in the fourth, key situational factors were good leadership and strong unit cohesion. Heroic soldiers were not the most obedient; some resistance to military authority appeared to foster heroic behavior. Overall, the study demonstrates that strong unit cohesion and good unit leadership elicit the best from soldiers in combat.

The studies undertaken by the Israelis following the 1973 war show that battle-shock can emerge very quickly if fighting is sufficiently intense; that delayed battle-shock can be a significant problem; that civilian stress, particularly family turmoil, can predispose to becoming a battle-shock casualty; that forward treatment is more successful than rear or civilian treatment; and that small-unit leadership and cohesion are important in maximizing performance in battle and minimizing psychiatric casualties.

On the basis of the analyses of their experience in 1973, the Israelis adopted the U.S. doctrine for treating combat psychiatric casualties: a brief rest near the front with a rapid return to the unit. They delineated the following principles: hold and treat briefly battle-shock cases as far forward as possible. Evacuate by ground ambulance, and not by helicopter, to ensure local evacuation and to maintain psychological proximity to the front. Organize in advance for the holding, treating, and returning to duty of battle-shock cases. Inform unit commanders to expect battle-shock casualties and to expect these casualties to return to the unit after brief treatment. Minimize battle-shock casualties by ensuring good unit morale, specifically cohesion and strong leadership, and ensuring stable family and community life. If immediate treatment near the front is unsuccessful and further evacuation is required, maximize the chance of eventual recovery and minimize the risk of chronic disability by evacuating to convalescent camps where military discipline is maintained. And finally, plan for accurate and relevant recordkeeping during wartime so that information can be gathered and later evaluated.

The IDF instituted several relevant organizationall changes after the

1973 war. A psychiatric team was assigned to each medical battalion at the division level. This team was to provide the first echelon of treatment for battle-shock. The team would hold battle-shock casualties for twenty-four to seventy-two hours. A second echelon of treatment was planned to be located in military camps in Israel, away from civilian hospitals. The soldiers treated there were to wear uniforms and to conform to military discipline. Activities were to include military drill, abreactive therapy, and sports. Maximum stay was to be two weeks. These camps were to provide strong expectation of return to duty, to avoid the demoralizing effects of a permissive civilian environment, and to provide therapy in the form of abreaction. The Israelis also planned to train their psychiatrists and psychologists—the bulk of whom were reservists—to treat battle-shock by means of brief forward treatment.

The 1973 Arab-Israeli War was the first war in which the Israelis sustained psychiatric casualties in significant numbers. These casualties emerged in the first hours and days of the fighting and where the battle was most intense. The casualties took the form of battle-shock rather than battle fatigue. The Israelis were unprepared to treat these casualties. All were evacuated to the rear; many were treated in civilian hospitals; and many became chronically disabled. On the basis of their experience, combined with their review of the literature, the Israelis planned future use of the U.S. doctrine for treating battle-shock: a brief rest near the front with a rapid return to the combat unit. During the war in Lebanon in 1982 these plans were put to the test.

BATTLE-SHOCK IN THE 1982 WAR IN LEBANON

The 1982 war in Lebanon differed qualitatively and quantitatively from the 1973 Arab-Israeli War. The 1982 conflict was fought at the time and in the manner chosen by the Israelis. It was fought on one front. Israeli preparation was thorough. The war engaged only a portion of the IDF and did not stress its logistic support. Reserve medical personnel, including mental health officers, received training in IDF medical doctrine and field operations prior to the war. Mental health officers were trained in the doctrine of forward treatment of battle-shock casualties and practiced the application of this doctrine in medical field exercises.

For the war in Lebanon, the IDF planned three axes of northward advance—western, along the coastal plain; central, along the spine of the Lebanon Mountains; and, if the Syrians intervened, eastern up through the Bekaa Valley. The Syrians did engage, and the IDF fought along all three axes. The advance along the coastal plain presented the problems of military operations in urban terrain, and the advance along the spine of the Lebanon Mountains and up through the Bekaa presented the problems of military operations in mountainous and broken terrain. These military operations were conducted from June 6, 1982, until the cease-fire at noon on June 11, 1982. There was a further period of fighting from June 21 to 26, 1982, when the IDF cut the Beirut-Damascus Road. Most of the IDF casualties, including the psychiatric casualties, were sustained during these two periods of active fighting.

Despite the excellent preparation by the IDF, the war was hard-fought. The Palestine Liberation Organization (PLO) units, fighting in the built-up urban areas along the coastal plain, evaded IDF envelopments, fought retrograde actions along the western axis, and retreated with the bulk of their personnel to Beirut. The Syrian commandos in the Lebanon Mountains, supported by regular Syrian forces, blocked the IDF advance along the central axis. Syrian armored forces in the Bekaa, while sustaining heavy casualties themselves, slowed the IDF advance along the eastern axis and caused many Israelis casualties.

During the period of June-December 1982, the IDF suffered 2,600 wounded and 465 killed in Lebanon (Table 5.1). Of the wounded, 80 percent were evacuated past the Advanced Medical Battalion (AMB) to Israel proper. These casualties were treated in Israeli civilian hospitals. Their injuries were not necessarily severe, but in the IDF Medical Corps there is pressure for rearward evacuation, preferably air evacuation. The pressure was a result of the mobility required of forward medical units. This mobility increased the difficulty of holding and treating psychiatric casualties forward within the division area.

During June-Decmeber 1982, the IDF sustained 600 psychiatric casualties (Shipler, 1983, and Table 2). This figure includes battle-shock (i.e., pure emotional reaction to the stress of battle); mixed syndromes (i.e., emotional reaction to the stress of battle combined with an underlying personality disorder); delayed psychiatric casualties (i.e., emotional reaction to the stress of battle and mixed syndromes following demobilization or while home on pass); and battle-shock and mixed syndromes in the wounded. Battle-shock and mixed syndromes in the

Table 5.1
Physical Casualties in Israeli Forces in Lebanon, June–December 1982

Adapted from Dolev, Personal Communication

Wounded in action (WIA)	2600
80% evacuated beyond level of medical battalion	
Killed in action (KIA)	465
50% severe head injury	
20% severe crush injury to body	
5% for other reasons beyond help	

Thus, approximately 75% were beyond help even with the most vigorous medical and surgical intervention

Table 5.2
Incidence of Psychiatric Casualties (Battle-Shock and Mixed Syndromes) in Israeli Forces in Lebanon, June-December 1982

Adapted from Shipler 1983; and Noy, Personal Communication

Psychiatric casualties including wounded with psychiatric symptoms	600
Wounded in action (WIA) with no psychiatric symptoms	2,600
Killed in action (KIA)	465
For the 1982 war in Lebanon, the ratio of psychiatric casualties (including wounded with psychiatric symptoms) to WIA	23:100
For the 1973 Arab-Israeli War, the ratio of psychiatric casualties (not including wounded with psychiatric symptoms) to WIA	30:100

wounded constituted 10 percent of the total number of psychiatric casualties. Battle-shock casualties were the bulk of the cases. The fact that some of the casualties who broke down at the front were diagnosed as other than battle-shock (e.g., mixed syndromes) probably is due to the diagnosing professional's inexperience rather than to variations in the clinical picture. For the IDF in Lebanon, the psychiatric to wounded casualty ratio was 23:100 (in actual numbers 600:2600). During the 1973 war, the ratio was higher, approximately 30:100. It appears that for an equivalent degree of combat stress, indicated by the relative number of wounded, psychiatric casualties in the IDF were lower during the 1982 war in Lebanon than during the 1973 war.

Ten percent of all psychiatric casualties occurred among wounded soldiers (Table 5.2). Psychiatric disturbances were found in both the lightly and seriously wounded. The brevity of the intense fighting in Lebanon and the rotation of soldiers out of combat after one or two battles may account for this. In the 1982 war, a wounded soldier was not much more rapidly removed from the combat zone than a non-wounded soldier: all IDF soldiers in Lebanon were "short-timers."

In addition to the psychiatric casualties at the front, psychiatric breakdown occurred in men who were home on leave or who had been demobilized. It is customary, tactical situation permitting, to give forty-eight hours home leave to units recently engaged in difficult actions. During the fighting in Lebanon, a number of units received such passes. Some soldiers, while home on pass, broke down and became psychiatric casualties. Their symptoms and signs were repetitive thoughts and images of the war, and crying, loss of appetite, and sleeplessness. The soldiers were unable to account for these symptoms except, in a general way, to relate them to the war. They were referred for treatment to the IDF Mental Health Clinic in central Israel. The soldiers' descriptions of their experiences in Lebanon revealed traumatic events or sequences of traumatic events preceding the emotional turmoil. In the opinion of IDF psychiatrists and psychologists, these soldiers' emotional reactions would have been less severe had they remained with their units in Lebanon. In their view, passes and rapid, temporary demobilization weakened soldiers' supportive ties with their units, reduced their ability to cope with their combat experiences, and thereby created psychiatric casualties of soldiers who would not otherwise have broken down. Inasmuch as the majority of these soldiers were home because their entire unit had been demobilized, IDF mental health personnel rejected the idea that the soldiers were primarily those sent on pass because their commanders recognized in them the signs of incipient breakdown or that the symptoms and signs developed because the soldiers were afraid to return to the front. Many such cases of delayed psychiatric breakdown were seen at the IDF Central Mental Health Clinic.

The clinical symptoms reported by psychiatric casualties in Lebanon were similar to those reported by American forces in World War I, World War II, and the Korean War, and by the Israelis during the 1973 war, but different from those reported by U.S. forces in Vietnam (Bar-On et al., 1983) (see Tables 5.3 and 5.4.) Pure battle-shock was characterized by anxiety, depression, sleep disturbance, and fear. Battle-shock casualties appeared in the first few days of combat, and cases continued to emerge as the fighting continued. In most cases, the soldiers who broke down had been engaged in heavy fighting and had gone without sleep for two or more days. These cases were more numerous where the fighting was intense and the physical casualties high. Tactical errors by commanders, being ambushed, or being hit by friendly fire increased their incidence. Immediately preceding events were intense combat, seeing friends or one's own commander wounded or killed, and one's own close escape from death.

Following the 1973 war, the IDF adopted the U.S. principles of forward treatment for psychiatric casualties. Prior to the war in Lebanon, the IDF Mental Health Department planned to treat psychiatric casualties forward at the level of the AMB. Each AMB supports a division and is located 2 to 20 kilometers to the rear of the fighting. The IDF had conducted education and training, including field excercises, for the forward mental health teams. Each five-member team consisted of one psychiatrist, one psychologist, and three other mental health officers, either psychologists or social workers. According to IDF plans, psychiatric casualties were to be seen first at the battalion aid station and, if they required more than an hour or two of rest, then they were to be evacuated by ground ambulance to the AMB. There, the forward mental health treatment team would hold casualties forty-eight to seventy-two hours before either returning them to their units or, if they were unimproved, evacuating them further rearward. The treatment was to consist of physical replenishment (water, food, and sleep) and supportive individual and group psychotherapy. The psychiatric casualties were treated as soldiers, were made responsible for

Table 5.3
Symptoms Reported by Psychiatric Casualties in Israeli Forces in Lebanon, June–September 1982

Adapted from Bar-On, Solomon, Noy and Nardi 1983

1.	Anxiety	56%
2.	Depressive affect	38%
3.5	Sleep disturbances	34%
3.5	Fear-diffuse, focused	34%
5.	Social estrangement, detachment	24%
6.	Conversive reactions	22%
7.	Crying	21%
8.5	Decreased appetite	19%
8.5	Headache	19%
11.	Exhaustion, fatigue	17%
11.	Psychomotor disturbances	17%
11.	Disturbing dreams, memories	17%
13.5	Tremors	13%
13.5	Confusion, concentration disturbances	13%
15.	Speech, communication impairment	12%
17.5	Dissociative states	11%
17.5	Irritability	11%
17.5	Explosive aggressive behavior	11%
17.5	Memory impairment	11%
20.	Noise sensitivity, startle	10%

their own maintenance, and were required to keep their personal weapons.

Many cases of battle-shock were sufficiently mild to be treated with an hour or two of rest at the battalion aid station and then to be returned to their units. No records were kept of these cases. The remain-

Table 5.4
Psychiatric Symptom Clusters in Different Wars, Both U.S. and Israeli

Adapted from Bar-On, Solomon, Noy and Nardi 1983

	U.S.			Israel	
	WW I	WW II	V'NAM	1973	1982
Anxiety		X		X	X
Depressive affect	X			X	X
Fear, diffuse/focused	X			X	X
Constricted affect			X		
Disturbing dreams		X		X	
Exhaustion, fatigue		X			
Decreased appetite		X			
Intestinal discomfort		X			
Headaches		X			
Startle reaction	X				
Sleep disturbance		X		X	X
Tremors	X				
Psychomotor changes	X			X	
Conversion reaction	X	X		X	X
Confusion	X				
Social detachment			X		X
Dissociation	X			X	
Antisocial			X		
Aggressive			X		
Substance abuse			X		

ing cases were evacuated beyond the battalion aid station, entered into the statistical records, and treated either forward at the AMB or rearward in Israel.

Despite the plan for forward treatment, not all psychiatric casualties were treated close to the front. Some were treated in central and northern Israel. This was due to a lack of awareness on the part of battalion surgeons of the importance of forward treatment and to the tactical situation in Lebanon where the terrain is hilly and the narrow roads run through steep-walled valleys. Military traffic moving forward toward the front made rearward ground evacuation difficult. Evacuation from the battalion aid station for both the wounded and the psychiatric casualties was therefore frequently by helicopter. Once on board a helicopter, casualties were flown directly back to civilian hospitals in Israel, bypassing the AMB. Psychiatric casualties were evacuated with the wounded, by ground or air—if by ground then to the AMB, if by air then to Israel. Approximately half of the psychiatric casualties reached the AMB, while half reached civilian hospitals in Israel. This assignment to air or ground evacuation was random. The IDF quickly realized that psychiatric casualties were surfacing at civilian hospitals and put into operation a second echelon treatment facility in northern Israel; treatment teams there were organized to provide brief treatment similar to that used forward. Thus, the treatment of psychiatric casualties offered a comparison of the effectiveness of forward and rearward treatments (Noy, Solomon, and Benbenishti, 1983). (See Table 5.5.)

The doctrine of forward treatment applied by the IDF for the first time during the war in Lebanon proved effective. A few aggressive teams returned 95 percent of battle-shock cases to duty with their units (Enoch et al., 1983). The method of one of the teams is representative (Enoch et al., 1983). Initially, they conducted an interview to establish where the soldier had been, what he had done, and what had happened to him. This interview was oriented objectively rather than toward thoughts and feelings. The team confirmed two of the observations made in previous wars. First, thoughts and feelings inevitably followed the description of the objective events. Second, just describing what had happened clarified events and reduced the emotional turmoil. The team allocated the next six to eight hours of treatment to physical replenishment (water, food, and rest). Then the soldier was given useful tasks to do and was invited to join in supportive individual and

Table 5.5
Results of Treatment of Psychiatric Casualties in Israeli Forces in Lebanon, June–September 1982

Adapted from Noy, Solomon and Benbenishti 1983

(First number in each pair total psychiatric casualties; numbers in ( ) are pure battle shock casualties)

	Returned to unit	Not Returned to unit
Forward treatment		
(2–5 Km from the front; or on the border)		
Break occurred at the front	60% (66%)	40% (34%)
Rearward treatment		
(central and northern Israel)		
Break occurred at the front	40% (46%)	60% (54%)
Break occurred at home following demobilization or while on pass	16% (11%)	84% (89%)

By Chi Square on actual numbers, groups differ (p .0001).

group psychotherapy. Next, the team arranged for comrades from the soldier's unit and for the unit commander to visit the soldier. Then the soldier himself was taken to visit the unit. In these ways, mutual confidence between the soldier and his unit was restored. When the soldier had recovered enough to return to the unit, the team would arrange for his comrades from his unit to pick him up. This team took advantage of its proximity to the front and to the soldier's unit to maximize expectation that he would return and to reinforce the soldier's links to his comrades and commander. The team observed that units were happy to receive the soldier back, confirming the finding from other sources that under stress group members prefer someone they know to someone they do not know, regardless of presumed competence. With respect to themselves, the members of the psychiatric team noted that, because of their proximity to the front, they were all afraid. However, sharing the dangers of combat with the soldiers being treated made them less reluctant to return a soldier to his unit. They noted that their fear was diminished to the degree that the AMB commander was competent in ensuring their supplies of gasoline and other essentials. When this was not the case, they became more afraid, hoarded supplies, and saw their clinical effectiveness decline. The team observed their tendency to overidentify with the soldier they were treating; to want to be the "good father"; and to protect their newfound "son" from harm. This difficulty was reduced through once-a-day staff meetings for the purpose of discussing cases, providing mutual support, and working through emotional conflicts (Enoch et al., 1983).

The Israelis observed that the psychiatric symptoms changed from the time the soldier broke down at the front to the time he arrived at the AMB (Bar-On et al., 1983). At the front, most soldiers suffering psychiatric breakdown complained of inability to perform—termed by the Israelis "the ticket out" of combat—whereas upon reaching the AMB they complained of difficulties with thoughts and feelings—termed "the ticket in" of treatment. The Israelis concluded that the severity of initial symtoms had little to do with prognosis for recovery; the most important indicator of a good prognosis was the soldier's labeling himself as healthy, taking initiative in his own care, in helping others, and in helping run the treatment team's area (Enoch et al., 1983).

A problem in the application of the doctrine of forward treatment during the war in Lebanon was the pressure for rearward evacuation at both the battalion aid station and the AMB. The battalion aid stations were moving frequently, and as a result the battalion surgeons evacuated everyone they could, wounded or not, rearward. If evacuation was by helicopter, the casualties were flown directly back to Israel, bypassing the AMB. Similar pressures for evacuation existed at the AMB. In one instance, a small group of psychiatric casualties at an AMB was "whisked away" by a medevac helicopter from the care of the division psychiatrist who was planning to hold them there for treatment. The IDF subsequently instituted several changes in policy. First, no helicopter pilot may accept an unwounded soldier on a medevac flight. Second, no unwounded soldier may be evacuated by either ground or air beyond the level of the AMB. In addition, the Mental

Health Department is conducting a series of lectures for battalion surgeons on the rationale for forward treatment of psychiatric casualties and the consequent need to interrupt rearward evacuation of these casualties. From this combination of changes in regulations and education of medical personnel, the IDF hopes that future psychiatric casualties will be held for forward treatment despite the pressure for rearward evacuation.

For those soldiers diagnosed as psychiatric casualties and treated forward at the AMB, 75 percent were sent back to their units within seventy-two hours. Some failed to reach their units for administrative reasons, and a few relapsed, leaving a net 60 percent returned to duty with their units. In contrast, for soldiers diagnosed as psychiatric casualties and treated in Israel proper, return to duty was only 40 percent (Noy, Solomon, and Benbenishti, 1983). (See Table 5.5.) One rear treatment unit was as successful as the average forward treatment team in returning soldiers to duty, possibly showing that the team's expectancy that the soldier would return to duty was more important than proximity to the front. For both forward and rearward treatment, the IDF found that the following factors predicted return: relative youth, being a combat soldier, and carrying a diagnosis of simple battle-shock (Solomon and Noy, 1983). See Table 5.6.

The majority of psychiatric casualties occurred in combat soldiers early in the war. Six months after the beginning of the war, 100 of the 600 psychiatric casualties were still in ambulatory therapy. Of the 600, 25 to 30 percent had received a psychiatric profile and as a result had been excused from any combat duties. Five had been discharged from the military.

Of the delayed psychiatric casualties, most were referred for outpatient psychotherapy. A few were referred to the rear treatment facility in northern Israel. Only 16 percent were returned to their units (Noy, Solomon, and Benbenishti, 1983). See Table 5.5. These delayed psychiatric casualties were similar to those observed by the IDF in the 1973 war. The occurrence of delayed psychiatric casualties provides further evidence of the importance of comradeship and unit cohesion in maintaining soldier effectiveness not only before and during, but after battle as well.

Of the 600 soldiers evacuated as psychiatric casualties, 60 required further institutional treatment after two to three weeks of combined first- and second-echelon psychiatric care (Margalit et al., 1983). See

Table 5.6
Factors Correlated with Return to Duty Following Psychiatric Breakdown in Israeli Forces in Lebanon, June–September 1982

Adapted from Noy and Solomon 1983

Factors positively correlated with return to duty:

  Forward treatment

  Younger

  Being a combat soldier

  Being diagnosed as suffering from battle shock

Factors showing no correlation with return to duty:

  Pre-war medical history

  Country of origin

  Performance predictor score

  Intelligence

  Education

  Motivation score (on induction)

  Type of service (regular or reserve)

Table 5.7. Soldiers unresponsive to the brief initial treatment were sent to the Combat Fitness Retraining Unit (CFRU). The CFRU was located on the grounds of a sports institute in central Israel. The staff included psychiatrists, psychologists, social workers, and sports coaches who had worked with psychiatric casualties during and immediately after the 1973 war. The guiding idea of the CFRU was a combination of "walking and talking." The treatment program consisted of abreactive individual and group psychotherapy, individual and group sports, and combat-oriented military training. The mental health personnel and the sports coaches participated in both the psychotherapy and the physical activity. The sixty patients came about equally from regular and reserve units; the majority were from combat units. The average stay was twenty-six days. Only five patients (8 percent) received medication, in all cases antidepressants. The CFRU was relatively successful. Of the regular service soldiers, 43 percent were returned to their units, and of the reservists, 38 percent were returned; (Table 5.7). After completing treatment at the CFRU, none of the men required further institutional care, and some were well enough to return to combat duty in Lebanon.

The soldiers treated in the CFRU were given a variety of psychometric tests, including the Minnesota Multiphasic Personality Inventory (MMPI). Psychosocial histories were also taken. The test results and the psychosocial histories were given to six mental health officers who diagnosed the men with regard to psychiatric pathology. They were unaware that the men were psychiatric casualties. These blind evaluators diagnosed 90 percent of the sixty soldiers as suffering from some form of character disorder (Segal et al., 1983). In contrast, the mental health officers at the front thought character disorders were present in only a small proportion of their battle-shock cases. This confirms the impression from other wars and armies that personality contributes lit-

Table 5.7
Combat Fitness Retraining Unit (CFRU), Third Echelon of Treatment of Battle-Shock Casualties in Israeli Forces in Lebanon, June–September 1982

Adapted from Margalit et al. 1983

60 patients (10% of total) were treated at the CFRU

Equally divided between reservists and regular soldiers

Most were from combat units

Stayed an average of 26 days

5 patients (8% of total) received tricyclic antidepressants

Regular service soldiers:

    43% returned to original unit
    57% reassigned to non-combat unit

Reservists:

    38% returned to original unit
    62% reassigned to non-combat unit

A number of soldiers went back to combat in Lebanon

tle to the risk of breakdown in combat but substantially influences prognosis once breakdown has occurred. Thus, once they have become psychiatric casualties, soldiers with character pathology seem less likely to respond to brief forward treatment and are overrepresented in the second and third echelons of treatment. A similarly poor prognosis was observed in soldiers with repressed personalities who suffered battle-shock during the 1973 war (Noy, 1978b).

The IDF studied the recurrence of battle-shock in soldiers who had broken down in the 1973 war (Solomon, Oppenheimer, and Noy, 1983). See Table 5.8. By June 1982, the IDF still had 600 of these on record. Of these 600, 40 percent were combat-ready by profile. By comparison, of a control group of 1973 veterans, 75 percent were combat-ready by profile. Thus, by June 1982, significantly fewer former psychiatric casualties were combat-ready by profile, implying a degree of vulnerability to life-stress or chronic disability. Of the former psychiatric casualties who were combat-ready by profile (approximately 240), 200 fought in Lebanon. The recurrence rate for this group of psychiatric casualties was 1 percent. The recurrence rate in the control group of 1973 war veterans was 0.5 percent, and the overall occurrence rate for psychiatric casualties for Israeli reservists in Lebanon was 0.67 percent. Thus, there was no discernible difference in psychiatric breakdown rates in Lebanon between those soldiers who had suffered previous breakdowns during the 1973 war and those who had served in the 1973 war but had not broken down. The IDF concluded that if a soldier was fit for combat duty by profile, a previous history of battle-shock would not place him at increased risk for future combat-related psychiatric breakdown.

Throughout the history of modern warfare, psychiatric casualties have risen as a function of battle stress. Battle stress is typically measured as number of casualties per combat duty. In past wars, using this measure, the greater the battle stress, the greater the number of psychiatric casualties, both absolutely and as a fraction of total casualties. The IDF studied this in greater detail during the war in Lebanon by defining battle stress independently of physical casualties. The IDF chose four battalions for a retrospective study; these four battalions fought during the early stages of the war in Lebanon (Noy, Solomon, and Nardi, 1983). See Table 5.9. The after-action reports of the four battalions were given to six military mental health experts for review. Each was asked to rank the battles fought on the basis of preparation,

Table 5.8
Recurrence of Battle-Shock in Israeli Forces in Lebanon, June–September 1982

After Initial Psychiatric Breakdown in the 1973 Arab-Israeli War

Adapted from Solomon, Oppenheimer and Noy 1983

By June of 1982 battle shock cases from the 1973 Arab-Israeli War still on record	600
Of the above cases:	
Combat ready by profile	40%
By June 1982 of the control group of 1973 Arab-Israeli War veterans:	
Combat ready by profile	75%
Recovered battle shock cases from 1973 serving in Lebanon	200
Recurrence of battle shock in Lebanon in battle shock cases from 1973	1%
Occurrence of battle shock in the control group of 1973 Arab-Israeli War veterans	0.5%
Overall risk of occurrence of battle shock for all Israeli reserve forces in Lebanon	0.67%

type of battle, adequacy of support, enemy resistance, and commander's relation to higher command. The experts doing the ranking were not informed of the number of physical and psychiatric casualties each battalion had sustained during the battles in question. On the basis of the rankings, the battalions were then ordered by the overall amount of battle stress they endured. There was high inter-rater reliability among the experts, with five out of the six agreeing completely. Of interest is the IDF's inclusion among the components of battle stress the trust by the battalion commander in his higher command and the degree of pressure, justified or otherwise, that he received from his higher headquarters. The overall ranking of the battalions in terms of the amount of battle stress was then compared to the actual number of physical and psychiatric casualties sustained. The battalion ranking on the basis of battle stress also ranked them on the basis of physical and psychiatric casualties, and the ratio of psychiatric to physical casualties (Table 5.9). In spite of the small sample of units involved, the data reinforce the idea that casualty rates and battlefield stress are closely related and that when stress is greater, the fraction of psychiatric casualties is larger.

The IDF found that other factors correlated with psychiatric casualty susceptibility in Lebanon (Solomon and Noy, 1983). See Table 5.10.

Table 5.9
Battle Stress as a Predictor of Battle-Shock, Israeli Forces in Lebanon, June–September 1982

Adapted from Noy, Nardi and Solomon 1983

```
Based on the battles of 4 battalions
Battles were ranked on intensity of battle stress by the following
factors:

  Preparation (enemy location, mission, false alarms, training)
  Battle (artillery, air attack, ambush, hostage, mine field)
  Support (tactical, logistics, material)
  Enemy resistance (strong, adequate, weak)
  Trust by commander in the higher command (unjustified pressure,
     some pressure, adequate support)

Overall ranking of battle stress for each battalion (ranked 1-4 most
to least difficult; rank given in 1st column) compared to psychiatric
and physical casualties and the ratio of the two (expressed as
number of psychiatric casualties per 100 physical casualties (KIA +
WIA)). The overall ratio of psychiatric casualties to physical
casualties (KIA + WIA) for the war in Lebanon was approximately
20:100.
```

	Physical Casualties (KIA + WIA)	Psychiatric Casualties	Ratio
1.	36	31	86:100
2.	23	9	39:100
3.	10	1	10:100
4.	12	0	00:100

One was age. Soldiers aged eighteen to twenty-one appeared the least vulnerable, and soldiers aged twenty-six to thirty, the most vulnerable. Other factors correlated with psychiatric breakdown were poor education, low motivation, and low intelligence, being a reservist, being of low rank, and being from a support unit. To a degree these factors were interrelated. In the IDF, low education, motivation, and intelligence led to assignment in a support unit, and in the older soldiers these factors are associated with low rank. In addition, serving as the control group for this study were the wounded. Because the IDF places its more intelligent and well-motivated soldiers in combat units where there is a higher probability of being wounded, it is likely that wounded soldiers as a group are above the IDF average for intelligence and motivation. Thus, the above findings, with the exception of those related to age, are provisional, pending comparison of the psychiatric casualties to a control group of age, rank, and military occupation-matched unwounded soldiers.

Morale has been described as the secret weapon of the IDF. Since its creation in 1948, the IDF has stressed the importance of morale in combat and the role of policy and practice in fostering it. The 1973 Arab-Israeli War raised the IDF's awareness of the psychological apsects of combat to an even higher level. This has resulted in the rapid development of the scientific appraisal of morale, leadership, and unit cohesion, and their relationship to combat effectiveness. Since the 1973 war, the IDF has deployed psychologists at the brigade and division levels to study these factors and to give practical advice to company, battalion, brigade, and division commanders on morale and the other psychological factors important in maintaining performance in combat. In principle, prior to combat, these psychologists measure morale on a company-by-company basis, and during combat, they accompany brigade and division commanders, providing advice on a variety of morale factors. In practice, as the criteria for selecting combat psychologists are stringent, there are not enough of them to allow them to serve all combat units. Even when deployed, they do not systematically survey morale in all combat companies. Despite these limitations, the IDF has done interesting studies of morale and its relationship to other personal and unit factors as described below.

Company morale correlates significantly with personal morale. In the spring of 1981, a survey was conducted of the morale of 1,200 IDF combat soldiers. The purpose of this survey was to identify the

Table 5.10
Ratio of Battle-Shock to Wounded by Age in Israeli Forces in Lebanon, June–September 1982

Adapted from Solomon and Noy 1983

Age	Battle shock: wounded
18-21	10:100
22-25	22:100
26-30	38:100
31-35	29:100
36-55	28:100

By Chi Square on actual numbers, groups differ (p .0000).

Other factors predicting breakdown (battle stress held constant; wounded soldiers as the control group):

Low education

Low motivation score (personality characteristics and attitude towards military service)

Low performance predictor score (intelligence, motivation, knowledge of Hebrew)

Reservist

Support unit

Low rank

components of both personal and company morale (Gal, 1983). See Table 5.11. The components of personal morale are trust in the company commander, confidence in one's own skills as a soldier, one's feelings about the legitimacy of the war, trust in one's weapons, trust in one's self, confidence in one's comrades' readiness to fight, the unit's cohesiveness, and the quality of one's relationship with one's commander. The IDF has found that the component of trust in one's weapons has become an increasingly important factor in personal morale over the last three decades. Also of interest is the IDF finding that when belief in the legitimacy of war declines, as it did in soldiers

Table 5.11
Correlations Between Morale and Other Variables in Israeli Forces, May 1981

Adapted from Gal (1983)

Personal morale	.55	Perceived company's morale
	.32	Relations with commanders
	.36	Unit's cohesiveness
	.24	Trust in company commander
	.27	Comrades readiness to fight
	.28	Legitimacy of war
	.34	Trust in one's self
	.24	Trust in weapons
	.23	Personal competence
Perceived company morale	.55	Personnel morale
	.47	Relations with commanders
	.41	Unit's cohesiveness
	.27	Trust in company commander
	.20	Comrades' readiness to fight
	.09	Legitimacy of war
	.21	Trust in one's self

N = 1200; all correlations are significant (p .05)

fighting in Lebanon, overall morale can remain high if soldiers maintain trust in their commanders.

Company and personal morale and readiness correlated with several other factors. In a study conducted on 1,500 soldiers during the third week of the war in Lebanon, the IDF found current company morale and readiness, and current personal morale, significantly correlated with company functioning during combat, company morale during combat, trust in the commander, and self-appraisal as a soldier. Negatively correlated with all of the above were dysfunctions caused by fear. Uncorrelated with the above were casualties among commanders, information before and during combat, talks with commanders, and appraisal of the enemy. Thus, it would appear that companies with high unit and personal morale will show high levels of trust in their commanders, will fight well, and will be less easily suppressed by enemy fire. In contrast, casualties among commanders, information supplied by commanders, or fear of the enemy have little relation to morale, to effectiveness, or to liability to suppression. Although the correlations in Table 5.11 are not exceptionally high, the trends appear meaningful.

Trust in the commander depends primarily on the competence of the commander, and only secondarily on his credibility and caring for soldiers. Using data obtained from thirty platoons (approximately 300 soldiers) during the third week of the war (Kalay, 1983), the IDF has refined the concept of trust in the commander, dividing it into three components: belief in the professional competence of the commander, belief in the credibility of the commander, and the perception of how caring the commander is for his soldiers. All three components are important ingredients of trust in the commander in garrison. In combat, however, belief in the commander's professional competence becomes the primary ingredient of trust. The soldier's perception of the professional competence of his commander is complex. It includes both the perception of the commander's overall professional competence and, more specifically, the perception of the care with which the commander tailors the missions he receives from higher command to the particular strengths and weaknesses of the men under his command. In addition, the personal example of the commander—his demonstrated confidence in himself, his soldiers, and the unit's weapons—were important components of commander competence and hence of overall trust. Also important in commander competence were good navigational skills, prior combat experience, and following the alert regulations. In the war in Lebanon, the IDF found that of the three factors of trust in the commander—professional competence, credibility, and caring for soldiers—perception of the commander's professional competence by the soldiers under his command correlated most highly with combat effectiveness. In general, the IDF has found morale an effective predictor of unit performance in combat.

The IDF used their morale measures to study the incidence of psychiatric casualties. Historically, in addition to battle stress, low morale, poor unit cohesion, and weak leadership have predicted psychiatric casualties in battle. The IDF found that company morale was negatively correlated with the incidence of psychiatric casualties. However, this study has a number of methodological difficulties. Specifically, psychiatric casualties were recorded on a battalion-by-battalion basis, whereas the morale measures (when available) were done on a company-by-company basis. Since, in any given battalion, there are three combat companies and one support company, morale measures, in addition to being unavailable for all the combat companies, are not available at all the support companies. Thus, the study needs to be redone once the psychiatric casualties are analyzed on a company-by-company basis. Within the limitations of the method outlined above, the preliminary results indicate that the higher the morale of a unit going into combat in Lebanon, the less likely the unit was to suffer psychiatric casualties. From the importance the IDF attaches to morale in active service and reserve units it can be inferred that high morale also correlates with increased combat effectiveness. Furthermore, in elite Israeli units in Lebanon (commandos and other special units), psychiatric casualties were zero in spite of the intense battles in which they participated, a finding consistent with the experience of U.S. forces in World War II.

Despite high morale and a good deal of attention given by command to morale and the factors maintaining it, the IDF still suffered relatively high rates of psychiatric casualties during the war in Lebanon. This may be for the following reasons. Fighting in urban areas posed special problems for IDF soldiers. Battle-shock cases often resulted from the surprise of fire coming from among civilians (including women and children). Moreover, the IDF may have evacuated to the rear soldiers who had quite normal fear reactions to combat. Finally, the war in Lebanon was so brief in its active phases that all soldiers may have in effect been "short-timers" and suffered from a form of "short-timer's syndrome."

CONCLUSION

Psychiatric casualties were a significant source of manpower loss for the IDF in the 1973 Arab-Israeli War and in the 1982 war in Lebanon. In the four weeks of the 1973 Arab-Israeli War, the ratio of psychiatric casualties to wounded in action was approximately 30:100. In the 1982 war in Lebanon, from June through September, the ratio of psychiatric casualties to wounded was 23:100. The majority of psychiatric casualties were cases of battle-shock (pure emotional reaction to the stress of battle), but some were mixed syndromes, involving, in addition to battle stress, a component of character disorder. In both wars, intense battle stress was the primary cause of battle-shock. In both wars, battle-shock cases emerged within hours of the beginning of hostilities and were most prevalent where the battle was most intense. In both wars, symptoms were typically anxiety, depression, fear, and sleep disturbance. These were the symptoms that were typical of the battle-shock observed in the Allied armies in World War I, World War II, and the Korean War.

In both the 1973 and 1982 wars, most battle-shock casualties occurred in combat units. As a fraction of total unit casualties, however, battle-shock cases were more common in support units and among reservists. In the 1973 war, high levels of civil stress appeared to predispose to breakdown as well. In the 1982 war, low morale, low intelligence, low motivation, and poor education also may emerge (pending further analysis) as predisposing to breakdown.

The 1973 war was the first war in which the IDF sustained significant numbers of psychiatric casualties. They had no doctrine for treatment. All battle-shock casualties were evacuated to the rear; only a few returned to their units during the war; many became chronically disabled. Following the 1973 war, the IDF adopted the U.S. doctrine of forward treatment. Using forward treatment, the IDF was successful in sending 75 percent of soldiers back to duty within seventy-two hours. For administrative reasons some of these soldiers never returned to their units, and a few soldiers relapsed. Overall, 60 percent of psychiatric casualties were returned to combat duty following forward treatment. In comparison to forward treatment, rearward treatment was significantly less effective, returning only 40 percent of soldiers to their units. This contrast in effectiveness between forward and rearward treatment is consistent with the lessons learned from World War I, World War II, and the Korean War: if a psychiatric casualty is evacuated beyond the division, he is much less likely to return. In addition to forward treatment, good prognostic factors during the war in Lebanon included the psychiatric casualties taking initiative during treatment, being relatively young, being from a combat unit, and carrying a diagnosis of battle-shock. Of the soldiers who had become psychiatric casualties in the 1973 Arab-Israeli War, those who fought in Lebanon in 1982 were at no higher risk for developing battle-shock than other IDF soldiers. Of the battle-shock casualties in 1982 who received forward and/or rearward treatment and failed to recover following either form of brief treatment, 90 percent appeared to have an underlying character disorder. This supports the finding from the 1973 war that, whereas no particular personality is at risk for breakdown, character disorders do affect prognosis for recovery once breakdown has occurred. Nevertheless, with further treatment focused on physical and mental rehabilitation, even soldiers with underlying character disorders showed improvement so that 40 percent returned to their units. In the 1982 war in Lebanon, as in the 1973 war, the IDF found that high unit morale correlated with increased combat effectiveness and decreased psychiatric casualty rates.

REFERENCES

Bar-on, R., Solomon, Z., Noy, S., and Nardi, C. (1983). *War related stress: an overview of the clinical picture in the 1982 conflict in Lebanon.* Paper presented at the Third International Conference on Psychological Stress and Adjustment in Time of War and Peace, Tel Aviv, Israel, January 2–6, 1983.

Enoch, D., Bar-on, R., Barg, Y., Durst, N., Haran, G., Hovel, S., Israel, A., Reiter, M., Stern, M., and Toubiana, Y. (1983). *An indigenous military community as a psychotherapeutic agent: specific application of forward treatment in combat.* Paper presented at the Third International Conference on Psychological Stress and Adjustment in Time of War and Peace, Tel Aviv, Israel, January 2–6, 1983.

Gal, R. (1978). *Characteristics of heroism.* Paper presented at the Second International Conference on Psychological Stress and Adjustment in Time of War and Peace, Jerusalem, Israel, June 19–23, 1978.

Gal, R. (1983). *Unit morale—the secret weapon of the Israel Defense Forces.* Paper presented at the Third International Conference on Psychological Stress and Adjustment in Time of War and Peace, Tel Aviv, Israel, January 2–6, 1983.

Goren, Y., Triest, J., Segal, R., Margalit, C., Wozner, Y., and Nardi, C. (1983). *Contribution of group therapy in short term third echelon treatment program for combat reactions with poor prognosis.* Paper presented at the Third International Conference on Psychological Stress and Adjustment in Time of War and Peace, Tel Aviv, Israel, January 2–6, 1983.

Kalay, E. (1983). *The commander in stress situations in IDF combat units during the "Peace for Galilee" campaign.* Paper presented at the Third International Conference on Psychological Stress and Adjustment in Time of War and Peace, Tel Aviv, Israel, January 2–6, 1983.

Margalit, C., Segal, R., Nardi, C., Wozner, Y., and Goren, Y. (1983a). *Combat fitness retraining unit (CFRU) for short treatment and rehabilitation of combat reactions with poor prognosis in the June 1982 conflict.* Paper presented at the Third International Conference on Psychological Stress and Adjustment in Time of War and Peace, Tel Aviv, Israel, January 2–6, 1983.

Margalit, C., Segal, R., Goren, Y., Nardi, C., and Wozner, Y. (1983b). *Individual psychotherapy in a rear echelon unit for the treatment of combat reactions with poor prognosis in the June 1982 conflict in Lebanon.* Paper presented at the Third International Conference on Psychological Stress and Adjustment in Time of War and Peace, Tel Aviv, Israel, January 2–6, 1983.

Nardi, C., Wozner, Y., Margalit, C., Segal, R., and Goren, Y. (1983). *Behavioral approach in a combat fitness retraining unit (CFRU) in the June 1982 conflict in Lebanon.* Paper presented at the Third International Conference on Psychological Stress and Adjustment in Time of War and Peace, Tel Aviv, Israel, January 2–6, 1983.

Noy, S. (1978a). *An integrative model of treatment for combat reaction.* Paper presented at the Second International Conference on Psychological Stress and Adjustment in Time of War and Peace, Jerusalem, Israel, June 19–23, 1978.

Noy, S. (1978b). *Stress and personality as factors in the casuality and prognosis of combat reaction.* Paper presented at the Second International Conference on Psychological Stress and Adjustment in Time of War and Peace, Jerusalem, Israel, June 19–23, 1978.

Noy, S., Solomon, Z., and Benbenishti, R. (1983). *The forward treatment of combat reactions: a test case in the 1982 conflict in Lebanon.* Paper presented at the Third International Conference on Psychological Stress and Adjustment in Time of War and Peace, Tel Aviv, Israel, January 2–6, 1983.

Noy, S., Nardi, C., and Solomon, Z. (1983). *Battle characteristics and the prevalence of combat psychiatric casualties.* Paper presented at the Third International Conference on Psychological Stress and Adjustment in Time of War and Peace, Tel Aviv, Israel, January 2–6, 1983.

Segal, R., Margalit, C., Reish, M., Zilberman, S., and Friedman, Y. (1983). *The contribution of combat physical fitness in a rear unit (CFRU) for the treatment of combat reactions with poor prognosis.* Paper presented at the Third International Conference on Psychological Stress and Adjustment in Time of War and Peace, Tel Aviv, Israel, January 2–6, 1983.

Shipler, D. (1983). The other Israeli casualties: the mentally scarred. *New York Times*, January 8, 1983, p. 2.

Solomon, Z., and Noy, S. (1983). *Who is at high risk for combat reaction?* Paper presented at the Third International Conference on Psychological Stress and Adjustment in Time of War and Peace, Tel Aviv, Israel, January 2–6, 1983.

Solomon, Z., Oppenheimer, B., and Noy, S. (1983). *Subsequent military adjustment of soldiers who suffered from combat reaction in the Yom Kippur war.* Paper presented at the Third International Conference on Psychological Stress and Adjustment in Time of War and Peace, Tel Aviv, Israel, January 2–6, 1983.

Steiner, M., and Neumann, M. (1978). *Traumatic neurosis and social support in the Yom Kippur war returnees.* Paper presented at the Second International Conference on Psychological Stress and Adjustment in Time of War and Peace, Jerusalem, Israel, June 19–23, 1978.

Wozner, Y., Goren, Y., Margalit, C., Nardi, C., Segal, R., and Triest, Y. (1983). *Behavioral dynamics of a short term residential setting for the rehabilitation of combat reactions with poor prognosis at the CFRU.* Paper presented at the Third International Conference on Psychological Stress and Adjustment in Time of War and Peace, Tel Aviv, Israel, January 2–6, 1983.

6

Future Directions of Military Psychiatry

FRANKLIN D. JONES

Although the psychology of warfare as an element in motivating the soldier to perform well under fire has been known from before the first millennium, the closer connection between the soldier's mind-set and his ability to withstand the horrors of the battlefield remained elusive until the era of modern war. Sun Tzu, the famous Chinese military thinker, first spelled out the psychology of the warrior five hundred years before the birth of Christ. However, it was not until the seventeenth century, and then unclearly at that, that military service as a cause of psychiatric debilitation was first hinted at. It was in the seventeenth century that the first descriptions of a modern category of psychiatric reaction to battle appeared in military medical records, with conditions of "nostalgia" recorded among fighting troops (Rosen, 1975).

Nostalgia, a condition found among soldiers characterized by a general sense of weakness and inability to concentrate and generally perform military tasks, was called "the Swiss disease" because it was first noted among Swiss mercenary soldiers in the seventeenth century who had been transported far from home to fight a war in which they had little personal investment. Later, in the eighteenth- and early nine-

---

The views of the author do not purport to reflect the positions of the department of the army or the department of defense (Para 4-3, AR-360-5).

teenth-century Napoleonic Wars, Larrey described the condition of nostalgia as a significant cause of military ineffectiveness among French troops. He also developed a relatively sophisticated approach for treating the problem, an approach that incorporated a number of elements found in the modern treatment of combat stress casualties (Jones, 1985a).

Nostalgia appeared again among soldiers on both sides of the American Civil War and accounted for significant loss of manpower on both sides. During this conflict, this psychiatric response to combat stress was also called "homesickness." Shortly after the Civil War, the concept of nostalgia gradually faded from the medical literature dealing with stress under fire, most probably as a consequence of the popularity of a new psychiatric nomenclature developed by Emile Kraepelin. The emergence of Freudian psychodynamics at approximately the same time also contributed to the decline in the use of nostalgia as a diagnostic category. Yet, the reality—by whatever other name—remained. This author found the concept quite useful in describing "disorders of loneliness" which emerged among American combat troops in Vietnam. Indeed, there is significant evidence that nostalgic casualties may have been the predominant form of combat stress casualty in Vietnam and probably contributed strongly to the high levels of drug and alcohol abuse found among American soldiers during that conflict. It may well have also contributed strongly to the pressure for withdrawal of American troops as more and more soldiers began to manifest nostalgic symptoms.

It was the Russian experience in their war against the Japanese in 1905 that provided the first truly modern description and diagnosis of combat stress casualties. A major category of stress reaction defined by Russian psychiatrists in that war was neurasthenia, a condition that has a remarkably close symptomology to what had earlier been called nostalgia. It was not until World War I, however, that the number of psychiatric casualties among Allied forces became so large as to constitute a major source of combat ineffectiveness in soldiers. In general, the symptoms manifested by psychiatric casualties in World War I tended to simulate genuine neurological injuries such as paralysis, blindness, and surdomutism. Accordingly, such symptoms were thought to be due primarily to physiological damage to the brain and nervous system. Common causes were thought to be "commotion" in the brain, brain contusions, microbleeding in the brain's interior, and "molecular derangement" of brain tissue (Laughlin, 1967). Because such symptoms were often associated with the shock and concussion caused by heavy indirect fire bombardments for hours on end, they were often lumped together into the general category of "shell shock."

As the war continued, however, evidence began to mount suggesting that the symptoms associated with shell shock were, in fact, not caused by the physiological disruption of the brain or nervous system, but were psychogenic in origin. Studies found that often such psychiatric symptoms were absent from wounded soldiers even though they had ruptured eardrums from concussive shock; that German prisoners of war under bombardment did not develop stress syndromes while their allied guards did; that autopsies revealed that a number of individuals suffering from severe symptoms often had no damage to their brains; and, finally, that there were positive signs of hysterical conversive and dissociative disorders in those suffering from shell shock. Thus, by the end of the war, few military psychiatrists retained their belief in the physiological origins of symptoms of shell shock and began regarding them as psychogenic reactions to severe stress. The Soviets persisted in the physiological approach throughout World War I and retained it through World War II. Even more to the point, recent Iranian casualties in the Iran-Iraq War have been diagnosed as suffering from symptoms induced by concussive shock and were labeled "explosion blow" casualties (Mohajer and Mottaghi, 1985).

PRINCIPLES OF COMBAT PSYCHIATRY

During World War I the Americans, drawing heavily on the extensive British and French experience with psychiatric casualties, developed the concept and procedures for "forward treatment" for psychiatric casualties suffered by the American Expeditionary Force (AEF). Dr. Thomas Salmon, an American military psychiatrist, laid down what have today become the basic principles of military psychiatry for dealing with neuropsychiatric casualties. Briefly, these principles are proximity, immediacy, and expectancy.

The first principle required that the soldier suffering from stress reactions be treated in proximity to the battlefront. The need to treat the soldier as close as possible to the front arose from the experience of the British. The British habit of evacuating their stress casualties back to England apparently resulted in the deepening of neurosis/psychosis which worked strongly against rapid and even eventual recovery. The second principle required that the soldier be treated as immediately as possible to prevent a deepening of his condition. Generally, such treatments—often administered at the battalion aid station—tended to be both brief and fairly simple. Such things as short periods of rest, a change of clothes, and food appeared to work miracles in bringing a soldier out of his symptoms. The third principle maintained that the soldier should know that his psychiatric reactions were not going to allow him to escape going back to the front. Thus, the principle of expectancy requried that the soldier be told and the expectation engendered in him that he would have to return to his comrades. It was feared that if soldiers were allowed to escape the stress of battle by developing certain psychiatric symptoms, the number of stress casualties would increase dramatically.

In order to support this system of treatment, the Americans worked out a plan for a three-tiered system of treatment. Psychiatrists were to be stationed at division, front, and rear areas where they would be responsible for administering psychiatric treatment and returning casualties to the fighting. A further aspect of this system was the establishment of a central evacuation clearing and screening point through which all casualties would flow. The object was to screen from the flow those individuals who could be treated without further evacuation and returned to duty rapidly.

World War I ended before the American plan could be attempted on a large scale. Worse, the lessons about the structure and function of the principles of combat psychiatry seemed to have become lost in the interwar period, perhaps under the impact of Freudian approaches to the problem which at that time were regarded as more modern and advanced. It would take almost the first three years of World War II before the American Army once again rediscovered the principles and practices it had evolved in World War I for dealing with psychiatric casualties. Fortunately, by the Korean War the procedure for treating psychiatric casualties had been permanently established so that by Vietnam they became the mainstay of treatment.

Although there are any number of divergencies from these principles and practices among the armies of the West, in essence all Western armies utilize the same principles of combat psychiatry—immediacy, proximity, and expectancy. To a great extent, all try to stop the flow of psychiatric casualties to the rear by thorough screening at lower levels, and all try to treat the soldier as close to the front as possible.

Although such things don't always work as well as planned, especially so when the number of physical casualties overburdens the system, on balance the principles remain.

Thus, if a system of military psychiatry is to function successfully in a battle environment, it will require four essential elements:

1. A safe place near the battle area (refuge).
2. A treating person (therapist of some sort).
3. Time for restoring physiological needs (rest).
4. A method for going back to the front (return).

The point is that each element is absolutely critical to any hope that psychiatric casualties might be successfully dealt with in any war. But each of these elements is jeopardized by the very nature of modern, high-intensity warfare which is the hallmark of today's armies.

CHARACTERISTICS OF MODERN WAR

From an historical perspective two main groupings of combat stress casualties may be distinguished in terms of the symptoms such casualties are likely to manifest. In all wars it seems true that the nature and type of casualties are directly related to the intensity of warfare experienced as measured by the number of combat deaths and woundings that occur and the increased probability of actually being killed. Table 6.1 presents the most frequent types of psychiatric symptoms occurring in a number of wars fought during the last five decades. War itself may, in general, be becoming much more intense and lethal as a function of weapons technology. Yet, in any given war it is by no means assured that all available technology will be employed or employed with the same degree of effectiveness. Thus, it is possible to talk about categories of war as distinguished by the type of psychiatric casualties that are likely to result in each type.

At one extreme one finds the type of psychiatric casualties that occur in intermittent, low-intensity conflicts. Soldiers exposed to combat of this type are likely to share the problems of anyone who leaves home for a long period and finds himself in an inhospitable environment. Soldiers in this type of war are likely to manifest symptoms of drug and alcohol abuse, disciplinary problems and infractions, and high

Table 6.1
Symptom Clusters in Various Wars

Symptoms	WW I	WW II	Vietnam	Arab-Israel Wars 1973	1982
Depressive affect	X			X	X
Fear: diffuse, focussed	X			X	X
Noise sensitivity	X				
Tremors	X				
Psychomotor disturbance	X				
Conversion reaction	X	X		X	X
Confusion, Aprosexia	X				
Dissociative states	X			X	
Anxiety		X		X	X
Nightmares		X		X	
Exhaustion, Fatigue		X			
Decreased appetite		X			
Gastrointestinal		X			
Headaches		X			
Sleep disturbances		X		X	X
Constricted affect			X		
Social estrangement			X		X
Discipline problems			X		
Explosive behavior			X		
Drug abuse			X		

rates of venereal disease. Pre-Vietnam era soldiers posted in garrison settings demonstrated many of these symptoms, and American soldiers stationed in similar settings in Korea and Europe continue to do so. Perhaps the penultimate example of a low-intensity conflict with resulting psychiatric casualties manifesting the symptoms noted above was the Vietnam War. The traditional principles of treatment used to deal with the psychiatric problems that emerged among soldiers in Vietnam appear to have been less effective with these types of casualties than one would have thought.

FUTURE DIRECTIONS

At the other extreme is the high-intensity, highly lethal, continuous combat of the type that characterized many (but by no means most) of the conventional battles of World War I and II. The clearest example of this type of war to date is, of course, the 1973 Arab-Israeli War. The tempo of warfare in this environment is marked by numerous combat pulses each day—anywhere from ten to twelve compared to the three or four that marked high-intensity combat of World War II—and warfare that is almost continuous in that it is fought day and night for weeks on end with almost no respite. Psychiatric casualties in this type of war almost always manifest some extreme form of anxiety and emotional exhaustion. Yet, paradoxically, it is in precisely this most intense, most continuous battle environment that, if applied correctly, the traditional principles and practices of combat psychiatry seem to have the most success in reversing the conditions of psychiatric casualties. Undoubtedly, there is a point in the severity and intensity of battle when the effectiveness of these principles will be of little or no avail, even if battlefield conditions allow their application.

Most modern armies of some size and complexity cannot ascertain with any degree of certainty just what kinds of wars they will be expected to fight. Sometimes, as in the case of Iran and Iraq, a military engagement that was expected to end in a matter of weeks endures for years with a resulting change in the conditions of the battlefield under which military psychiatry is expected to function. As a practical matter, then, modern military forces must be prepared to operate in conditions ranging from long-range, low-intensity conflicts to sudden and moderately protracted, highly intense, and lethal environments. In general, if combat psychiatry can develop approaches that succeed in each of these extreme environments, then any combat environment that falls between the extremes ought not to present any appreciable problem as far as treating psychiatric casualties is concerned.

LOW-INTENSITY FUTURE WARS

As a general rule, none of the major military powers of the world is likely to engage in a war characterized by an exchange of nuclear, chemical, and biological weapons. At least this would seem to be an article of necessary faith since such a war would be so destructive in all its dimensions as to make any consideration of how to treat psychiatric casualties—or any other casualties for that matter—almost a minor question. It is much more likely that the major powers will engage in the long-range, low-intensity conflict that was characteristic of Vietnam or of the Soviet intervention in Afghanistan. Less likely, yet still a distinctly realistic probability, is the type of warfare that characterized the Arab-Israeli conflict of 1973.

If the Vietnam experience is instructive (data from the Afghan War are almost toally lacking), it is likely that any future low-intensity conflict will produce precisely those nostalgia-like psychiatric casualties that emerged in Vietnam. Table 6.2 presents the characteristics of such casualties in terms of the precise types of symptoms they are likely to manifest. The data in the table also address those conditions that help aggravate and ameliorate the manifestation of nostaglic casualties. Generally any army attempting to sustain itself in a low-intensity combat environment must find ways to strengthen those conditions that ameliorate nostalgic casualties. Accordingly, ways must be found to minimize the family stress of the soldier, to enforce vigorous discipline in organized camp conditions, and, perhaps most important, to promote and enhance the degree of social cohesion that the soldier manifests toward his peers, his NCOs, and his officers. At the same time, of course, ways must be found to lessen the impact of those conditions that aggravate nostalgic casualties. Thus, ways must be found to prevent boredom in the long periods between actual combat engagements, to prepare the soldier to deal with extreme cultural differences that might affect the way he sees his role in the war, and to strengthen the social support of his peer groups, his family, and his nation.

Such things are much easier said than done. Indeed, if history is any guide, it seems clear that one can conclude that if a nation is going to fight this kind of long-range, low-intensity war, one ought not to use draftees in such campaigns. The professional soldier seems better geared to deal with the psychological conditions encountered in a low-intensity environment with a strange culture. If the Vietnam experience showed anything, it was that draftees do not function well psychologically in such environments, although it did not show that professional soldiers do that much better. In any case, it seems reasonable that most major military powers have the military manpower resources to select from their populations proper types of soldiers to at least fight the initial stages of a low-intensity conflict. Whether they have the foresight and political maneuverability to do so, however,

Table 6.2
Factors and Characteristics of Nostalgic Casualties

Aggravating Conditions

>   Initial Separation from Home
>   Dependant Personality Traits
>   Family Stress
>   Breakup of Dyadic Love Relationship ("Dear John" Letter)
>   "Culture Shock"
>   Boredom
>   Disorganized Camp Conditions
>   Inclement Weather
>   Static Warfare or Reverses in Combat
>   Anticipated Defeat or Prolonged Warfare
>   Lack of Friends in Unit

Ameliorating Conditions

>   Prior Separations Handled Successfully
>   Independent Personality Traits
>   Absence of Family Stress
>   Intact or Absent Dyadic Love Relationship
>   Dislocation to Similar Milieu
>   Rigorous Discipline
>   Organized Camp Conditions
>   Clement Weather
>   Victorious Battles
>   Anticipated Victory or Brief War
>   Multiple Friends in Unit

Characteristics of Nostalgic Casualties

>   Consticted Affect
>   Social Estrangement
>   Disciplinary Problems
>   Explosive Aggression
>   Substance Abuse
>   --------------------------------------
>   Sexual Problems
>   Post-Traumatic Stress Disorders
>   Delayed Post-Traumatic Stress Disorders

Source: Jones 1984a

remains quite another matter as does a power's ability of seeing the conflict through to its conclusion.

Thus, whereas low-intensity warfare is far more likely to occur than high-intensity conflict, its military consequences are not likely to be as drastic. Moreover, the tempo of development is likely to be considerably more gradual—as it was in Vietnam—so that the treatment of psychiatric casualties is not likely to be a major problem, at least not in terms of suddenly depleting the manpower pool of available military resources. It is high-intensity wars that present the real problem for military psychiatry.

HIGH-INTENSITY FUTURE WAR

Having had minimal recent experience in high-intensity warfare, most Western military forces must prepare for levels of combat of unprecedented ferocity, lethality, and destructiveness of conventional combat. If the enemy is the Soviet Union, then Western military forces will indeed face a type of warfare for which historically they are totally inexperienced. Soviet doctrine as it addresses a NATO-Warsaw pact confrontation calls for continuous military operations, including massed multi-echeloned assaults with armored, airborne, airmobile, and mechanized infantry units. Soviet assaults will be coordinated with massed artillery fires of heretofore unwitnessed proportions to include the use of limited nuclear and chemical weapons. Soviet units, especially the Operational Mobile Groups, will be expected to penetrate NATO defenses in great depth ranging up to 150 miles in the NATO force rear, disrupting communications and resupply activities. Soviet plans also call for a continuous assault by taking maximum advantage of their superior numbers and fighting at night. While they will attempt to rotate their units out of the line for short periods of rest, in practice, Soviet units will be fought down to 30 percent of strength, as they were in World War II, before they can expect rotation to the rear. In cases where the Soviet attack meets unexpected resistance, units will fight until they can no longer perform. Even then, these units will not be rotated out but will instead be seconded to replacement units so that the enemy resistance can be overcome. In the attack, Soviet units will also be seconded to new units in order to keep the tempo of the attack on schedule. NATO forces, by contrast, will be thrown on the defensive, with only a minimum depth defensive belt to their rear. Even this will be under continuous attack as Soviet units which break through the defensive lines roam almost at will in the rear areas. Resupply to forward units will be difficult, if possible at all, and NATO units will be forced to remain engaged with enemy forces almost continuously. The level of mental and physical stress will reach tremendous levels for very long periods of continuous combat.

Despite their planned use of weapons of mass destruction on the battlefield, the Soviets are fully aware of the psychological factors in the equation of combat effectiveness. By taking the offensive, most probably coupled with a strong element of tactical surprise, the Soviets fully intend to maximize the psychological impact of their attacking units. Soviet attacking forces calculate their hitting power not only in terms of physical casualties they expect to inflict, but also in terms of precise numbers of psychological shock casualties they can bring about. Soviet tactical manuals have calculated the shock effect—as opposed to the killing effect—of various types of weapons and units deployed in various ways in precise terms. One major goal of the forward edge Soviet attacking units is not so much to kill as to shock defending units so that they can bring about a state of what they call "battlefield paralysis." In the Soviet view, battlefield paralysis is induced by shock of attacking units wherein specified numbers of defending units are unable to effectively use their weapons. For example, a Soviet regiment firing one unit—of artillery can expect to paralyze the defenders for a period of 30 seconds to 5 minutes, depending on the type of weapon and unit affected. This period of time will allow echeloned Soviet units to close rapidly behind their barrage and attack with smoke and flamethrowers passing quickly through the defending unit and continuing the assault. The second echelon force will then deal with the remnants of the overrun units, while the first echelon continues to press the attack in the enemy's rear. Once in the enemy's rear, Soviet units will attempt to disrupt the defender's command, control, communications, petroleum depots, airfields, and other tactical and stratetic assets. In short, the Soviet attack plan is for a massive multi-echeloned combat pulse which can shock and disrupt the enemy in enough depth to permit the full deployment of its greater forces and to do it quickly. In general, the Soviets are planning for no more than a sixty-day war in Central Europe and fully expect to spend almost half that period mopping up pockets of isolated enemy resistance.

With regard to the use of tactical nuclear weapons—if, indeed, such things can be seriously said to exist when deployed over the large urban population concentrations of Central Europe—the Soviets see their use in very practical terms. They seem to believe that such weapons will be forced into use anyway as a consequence of the dynamics of the battlefield. No doubt, they feel that their employment in the larger offensive is a vital weapon in directly influencing the outcome of the battle. As a practical matter, NATO planners assume as a matter of course that the Soviets will use such weapons. If such weapons are used in the first minutes of the attack, the Soviets can reasonably expect to catch NATO forces either in garrison or in the process of mobilization. If NATO forces are on alert, the Soviets intend to use their intelligence and overflight capabilities to locate NATO units—focusing particularly on command and control headquarters—and to strike them quickly. In the end, of course, the battlefield will come to resemble the mobile front of World War II, only with increased lethality and stress that might surpass that of World War II combat by a factor of ten. The characteristics of such a high-intensity war appear in Table 6.3.

Under such terrible battle conditions, how effectively will the traditional principles of military psychiatry operate? Table 6.4 presents data showing that in such an intense and lethal environment of combat, military psychiatry cannot function in any meaningful way. In the first place, there will be no safe forward areas where psychiatric casualties can be treated. Technology has made such locations functionally obsolete. At a minimum, the employment of weapons systems capable of discovering aggregations of personnel through the infrared signatures given off by groups of soldiers and their supporting machinery (trucks, generators, and so on) will make such holding areas highly vulnerable. Moreover, even the geographic stability required by such areas will disappear as the front moves to the rear as attacking forces penetrate the defensive area. Furthermore, in such a war attacking forces may well bypass defensive strong points, preferring to penetrate into the soft rear areas where maximum damage can be inflicted at rapid rates of penetration, with little in the way of significant casualties proffered upon attacking forces. In short, attacking and defending forces and positions will merge into a giant miasma of movement, death, and destruction. There will be no safe places to treat psychiatric casualties near the front.

Even if methods are found to protect such areas from enemy penetration, the time needed to restore the soldier's physiological and emotional needs will be too short to make the return of the soldier to his original unit a practical probability. It is assumed, of course, that his original unit exists in sufficient force to make returning him to it

Table 6.3
Characteristics of High-Intensity Warfare

High Lethality with Mass Casualties
    "Disaster-Fatigue" Casualties

Continuous Combat
    Sleep Deprivation
    Increased Fatigue

High Mobility
    Radar Localization
    Proportionally Fewer Forces

Dispersal of Forces
    NBC Threat
    Infrared/Radar "Signature"
    Result of High Mobility

Absence of Air Superiority
    Limited Helicopter Medical Evacuation

Absence of Rear Battle Free Area
    Limited Traditional Medical Treatment

Source: Jones 1984b

Table 6.4
Negation of Principles of Forward Treatment

No Refuge:	Absence of Rear Battle-Free Area
No Therapist:	Dispersal of Forces Mass Casualty Situation (Triage)
No Rest:	Absence of Rear Battle-free Area High Mobility Lack of Time to Treat
No Return:	Dispersal of Forces High Mobility

Source: Jones 1984b

worthwhile to begin with. During World War II, the Soviets found that attempting to return soldiers to their units was not worthwhile, for, in their absence, the chances were too great that the unit had suffered such severe casualties as to make it combat ineffective. The Soviets responded to the problem by abandoning any attempt at unit replacement, opting instead for an individual replacement system built around replacement depots. Moreover, it is unlikely that it will be possible to return recovered psychiatric casualties to their units inasmuch as they must remain dispersed and in constant motion to avoid being detected by enemy intelligence systems and thus targeted for destruction. Yet, the evidence from World War II and Korea suggests that a soldier who once becomes a psyhciatric casualty, recovers, but cannot be returned to his unit is at great risk of becoming a psychiatric casualty again. Finally, it is unlikely that any system of air evacuation will be able to operate with any degree of effectiveness in the NATO rear areas, making it highly problematic that it will even be possible to evacuate psychiatric casualties from whatever holding points might exist.

Surgical and psychiatric casualties in a high-intensity battle scenario are expected to occur in such large numbers that medical personnel will be forced to use triage principles and practices developed for mass casualty disaster situations. Triage emphasizes treating first those casualties who have the best chance of survival and postponing treatment of those more seriously wounded or incapacitated. In any triage situation such as this, physical surgical casualties will have priority over psychiatric casualties—especially in the allocation of medical personnel resources—even though it is the stress casualties who are most likely to be able to become effective with minimal intervention. The Soviets themselves encountered this situation many times during World War II, and they always resolved it in favor of surgical casualties. At the very least, the full range of shock symptoms—paralysis, surdomutism, blindness, fugue states, conversion psychosis, and so on—which has been witnessed in other wars can be reasonably expected to emerge again, only this time among far greater numbers of men and with far greater military effect.

In essence, then, the expected battlefield conditions of a high-intensity conflict will virtually preclude the ability of the more traditional approaches of dealing with psychiatric casualties from working with any degree of effectiveness. In one swoop, modern war seems to have gone a long way to increasing the number of psychiatric casualties it will generate, while, at the same time, making it highly improbable that fighting armies will be able to deal effectively with psychiatric losses. Worse, unable to effectively deal with psychiatric casualties, this in itself becomes yet another problem which the military force must somehow manage. How is this to be done?

NEW PRINCIPLES OF COMBAT PSYCHIATRY

Because high-intensity warfare is likely to make the implementation of the traditional principles and practices of military psychiatry unworkable, new principles of combat psychiatry must be developed. Repeated studies have shown that psychiatry casualties occur in direct proportion to the intensity of combat and certain physical and morale factors. Factors tending to prevent psychiatric breakdown include reduced fatigue, presence of good small-unit leadership in which soldiers have confidence, confidence of soldiers in their weapons and themselves, attacking rather than defending, and a strong sense of unit social cohesion. Yet, the conditions of modern high-intensity warfare, with its high rates of surgical casualties, high mobility, widespread unit dispersion, and almost continuous quality, all work against reducing psychiatric casualties.

In the 1973 Arab-Israeli War, the only relatively recent example of high-intensity warfare, some of these factors were not appreciated. The hastily assembled Israeli units went into battle with less unit cohesion than their more stable counterparts. Moreover, these already weakened units were exposed to conditions of warfare for which they were not adequately prepared. The result was very high rates of psychiatric casualties. Available estimates of acute psychiatric casualties among Israeli forces expressed as a percentage of total casualties range between 30 and 50 percent! According to Egyptian military psychiatrists, the Egyptian psychiatric casualty rate at least equaled their rate of surgical casualties (Mansour, 1982), that is, they were at least 50 percent.

After the war, the Israelis made a concerted attempt to prevent future psychiatric casualties by establishing a psychiatric treatment and preventive structure modeled along the lines of that found in the U.S. military. Yet, when Israeli forces went into battle again in the 1982 incursion into Lebanon, the psychiatric casualty rate again proved to be very high, accounting for some 23 percent of total combat casualties, most of which occurred during the first two weeks of active combat (Belenky and Jones, 1983). It appears likely, then, that armies must either be prepared to treat large numbers of psychiatric casualties—a condition mitigated against by the very nature of the high-intensity warfare which generates such large numbers of psychiatric casualties—or find more effective ways to prevent them from occurring in the first place. What is needed is no less than a completely new set of principles of combat psychiatry. An overview of such principles is displayed in Table 6.5.

PREVENTION

Historically, armies have sought to prevent the occurrence of psychiatric casualties by screening the manpower pool, usually conscripts, in order to locate and remove from battle exposure those individuals which extant psychiatric screens have a priori defined as vulnerable to breakdown. The American Army attempted this process in World War

Table 6.5
Principles of Combat Psychiatry in High-Intensity Warfare

Prevention:

    Unit Cohesion
    Realistic Training
    Doctrine of Rest and Nutrition

Battlefield Treatment:

    Limited Evacuation of Psychiatric Casualties
    Treatment in the Midst of Battle
    Emphasis on Buddy Care: Reassurance
                              Expectancy

Use of Drugs:

    Non-sedating Anti-anxiety Drugs
    Non-depleting Stimulants to Reduce Fatigue
    Reversible Sleep and Alerting Agents

Source: Jones 1984b

II with disastrous results. The screening procedure obviously took on a life of its own and resulted in some 504,000 men—enough manpower to staff fifty combat divisions—being released from combat units as a result of one sort of psychiatric debilitation or another. The screening procedure failed in another sense. Although American combat forces had been repeatedly screened to remove vulnerable soldiers from battle, once American units were committed to the fighting, the overall rate of psychiatric debilitation still reached thirty-six per thousand, a rate considerably higher than American forces had suffered in World War I and much higher than that suffered by Soviet and German forces in World War II.

The failure of the screening process was compounded by a failure to understand the "chronology of breakdown," the time-bound process through which most soldiers pass on the way to becoming psychiatric casualties. The chronology of breakdown was not fully described until 1946, after the war was over. Swank and Marchand's work on the subject suggested that there were two distinct groups of soldiers that were prone to becoming psychiatric casualties: those never exposed to combat and those exposed to combat for a prolonged period of time. It is possible to chart the efficiency and vulnerability of both groups, measuring efficiency of action against time of exposure to combat. In the period of initial exposure, combat efficiency is low and the potential for becoming a psychiatric casualty is relatively high. After about three weeks of exposure, the soldier becomes somewhat accustomed to battle, and combat efficiency increases as vulnerability to breakdown declines. After five to seven weeks of exposure to combat, however, combat efficiency again begins to decline, this time drastically, while the vulnerability of the soldier to psychiatric breakdown increases rapidly. Moreover, there is no such thing as "getting used" to battle. With sufficient exposure to combat—on average about five to seven weeks—almost all men will eventually become psychiatric casualties of one sort or another.

Using the experience obtained during World War II, the American Army attempted to prevent psychiatric casualties by the simple expedient of reducing the amount of time the soldier would be exposed to the combat environment. Thus, in Korea and again in Vietnam, American soldiers were exposed to limited combat tours. Instead of being in service "for the duration," soldiers were limited to a nine-month tour of combat service in Korea and one year in Vietnam. More recently, the American military has focused on preventing high rates of psychiatric debilitation on the part of "green troops." On balance, this program seems to imitate the Israeli program of enhancing cohesion based on the findings of a number of studies showing combat proficiency to be related to cohesion. Thus, programs have been undertaken to increase cohesion by limiting officer and NCO rotational turbulence, keeping units together from Basic Training through overseas deployment, increasing training to instill further confidence in the soldier's ability to use his weapons, and providing more exposure to live-fire training exercise. It remains an open question for all armies whether the realities of the battlefield can be blunted by increasing unit cohesion. In his work, *The Face Of Battle*, Keegan suggests strongly that modern high-intensity war is so destructive and so rapid that attempts to deal with it by increasing unit cohesion will meet with only marginal success.

TREATMENT ON THE BATTLEFIELD

Any new principles of treating psychiatric casualties in battle must meet the test of working amid the environment of high-intensity warfare, something that cannot be approximated in training. Nonetheless, given what we know about high-intensity combat, it seems clear that new principles are needed. A first new principle of combat psychiatry would be to severely limit the evacuation of psychiatric casualties in order to prevent the rise of large-scale "evacuation syndromes" on the part of stressed soldiers. The Israelis have already made some moves in this direction, however tentative, by refusing to evacuate by helicopter any soldier who does not have an obvious physical wound. The intent is to prevent the evacuation of purely psychiatric casualties. Under this system, many of the psychiatric casualties would be held on the line.

A second principle would be to have the psychiatric casualty treated by his fellow soldier, his unit or element commander, or medical aidsman on the spot. The Soviets used this system to great effect in World War II, evacuating far fewer psychiatric casualties than most armies of the West while returning far more potential psychiatric casualties to the fighting. The Soviet military still espouses this doctrine of immediate soldier aid in its doctrine of "self-help for the soldier" in which the soldier is told that if he cannot help himself or receive help from his buddy, he might be left behind. The presence of a political officer in each Soviet company provides a treatment person whose main task is to keep the soldiers fighting by dealing with psychiatric casualties on the spot. The actual treatment that a soldier would receive under the new principles of combat psychiatry would consist of reassurance from his peers, the expectancy that he must remain on the line or suffer a worse fate, and possibly, at some time in the future, the administration of some nonsedating anti-anxiety drugs (Jones, 1985a). For the soldier who appeared severely fatigued or depressed, nondepleting stimulants would be administered. A nondepleting stimulant is one that does not deplete the nerves of the neurotransmitters. Such depletion which occurs, for example, with amphetamines eventually results in rebound fatigue and depression. The amino acids L-tyrosine and L-phenylalanine may be considered nondepleting stimulants.

DRUGS IN COMBAT

The most consistent symptom of combat stress, whether it occurs early in exposure to combat or after cumulative exposure, is anxiety. Anxiety may be manifested as fear, hysterical conversion or dissociation, tremors, or similar symptoms as outlined in Table 6.1. In the past, drug treatment of anxiety with sedatives, ranging from chloral hydrate and bromides in World War I to barbiturates in World War II and even self-prescribed drugs like alcohol, cannabis, and heroin in Vietnam, not only produced unwanted sedation of the soldier but also decreased the probability of the soldier's return to battle owing to the fixation of a sickness role suggested by taking medication. Indeed, based on their experience in the 1973 war, the Israelis have prohibited the forward use of medications and even hypnosis.

The problem is to find a drug that will selectively reduce the soldier's anxiety without diminishing his mental or physical alertness and efficiency. To some extent this occurred in the Vietnam War when physicians treated the psychophysiological symptoms of fear and anxiety with neuroleptics, that is, major tranquilizers, antipsychotics, and anti-anxiety agents (Datel and Johnson, 1981). The ideal drug to treat or prevent combat stress breakdown would be an easily administered, stable compound that would prevent development of or remove anxiety without producing significant neuromuscular or cognitive impairment. Such a drug would also have to be nonaddictive and permit the soldier's mind and body to respond appropriately to sudden danger. Unfortunately, such a drug is not currently available, but research continues.

Other drugs for selected purposes may also be developed. A drug with short duration of effect which is readily reversible by an antagonist could prove to be a most useful battlefield hypnotic. Such drugs are already in the experimental stage (Paul, 1982). Other studies suggest that buspirone may relieve anxiety without significant cognitive impairment in both acute and chronic use.

In sum, the development of such combat drugs may be the modern equivalent of an age-old practice found in combat armies. For centuries, fighting men have been given—or taken on their own—a number of "drugs" to enhance combat performance and relieve the stresses of war. Such drugs range from the British military's practice of giving the soldier a jigger of rum before battle, to the Soviet practice in World War II of having their paratroopers drink tea or coffee to "open the pathways to the brain," to the use of hashish by Ottoman Egyptian soldiers, or to the use of peyote by American Indian warriors, all designed to prevent or control fear. With the "revolution in psychopharmacology" which began in France in the early 1950s, the time may now be opportune for the use of drugs specifically designed and tailored to control fear and anxiety in combat.

CONCLUSION

Warfare has changed, perhaps forever. One cannot, after all, "disinvent" certain kinds of weapons, and there is no evidence to suggest that humankind has evolved to the point where the increased horror of weapons makes their employment any less likely than in the past. Indeed, it is precisely their newly acquired technological horrific effects which recommends their employment much more readily than in the past. Somehow, amid all this, the soldier must stand and fight. Somehow, he must convince himself that it all makes sense and that there remains some connection between his own actions and the probability that he will survive the storm of horror even when statistical studies of war suggest there is no truly functional connection at all.

In the effort to stand and do his duty, the soldier runs a great risk that he will be unable to remain sane, and that his psychological and physiological defenses will crumble with amazing rapidity. If war will not go away, and it seems certain that it won't, then some way must be found to deal with the terrible human fragility that the soldier brings to his environment of battle. Somehow, modern armies must cope on the human level with the effects of war that they have brought into being on the technological level.

Yet, the realities remain. Even with a revolution in the principles and applications of military psychiatry, the reality is that the new approaches outlined here would serve to reduce the chances that the soldier would be relieved from the horrors of combat even when he had reached his human breaking point, even after he had given all he could possibly give by any reasonable human standard. Worse, the amount of treatment that he could reasonably expect of trained psychiatric physicians would be reduced, throwing yet another burden on the soldier and his peers to treat themselves. Such conditions, inevitable though they might eventually become, would likely mean increased numbers of psychosomatic casualties, misdiagnosis of many suffering from breakdown, and, perhaps cruelest of all, an increased death rate even among treated cases of psychiatric breakdown. Perhaps, in the end, Keegan is correct when he says that war has become too horrible for the human mind and body to realistically tolerate. Even so, since war will not be abandoned by the human species in any forseeable future, the need to cope with these realities remains as strong as ever. Perhaps, even stronger.

REFERENCES

Appel, J. W., and Beebe, G. W. (1946). Preventive psychiatry. *Journal of the American Medical Association*, *131*, 182–189.

Aubin, S. P., and Kels, R. E. (1985). Airland battle doctrine: Soviet strategy revisited. *Military Review*, 65 (10), 42–53.

Bailey, P., Williams, F. E., and Komora, P. O. (1929). *The Medical Department of the United States Army in the World War*: Volume 10. *Neuropsychiatry*. Washington, D.C.: U.S. Government Printing Office, pp. 1–12.

Bar-on, R., Solomon, Z., Noy, S., and Nardi, C. (1983). *War related stress: An overview of the clinical picture in the 1982 conflict in Lebanon*. Paper presented at the Third International Conference on Psychological Stress and Adjustment in Time of War and Peace, Tel Aviv.

Belenky, G. L. (in press). Varieties of reaction and adaptation to combat experience. *Bulletin of the Menninger Clinic*.

Belenky, G. L. (1985). *Combat reaction spectrum disorder*. Paper presented at the annual meeting of the American Psychiatric Association, Dallas.

Belenky, G. L., and Jones, F. D. (1983). *The Lebanon experience: lessons of the Arab-Israeli war*. Paper presented at the William C. Menninger Memorial Conference entitled "Military Psychiatry and Stress." Proceedings in press, Topeka, Kansas.

Belenky, G. L., Newhouse, P., and Jones, F. D. (1982). Prevention and treatment of psychiatric casualties in the event of a war in Europe. *International Review of the Army, Navy and Air Force Medical Services* (Paris), *55*, 303–307.

Belenky, G. L., Tyner, C. F., and Sodetz, F. J. (1983). *Israeli battle shock casualties: 1973 and 1982* (WRAIR Report NP-83-4). Washington, D.C.: Walter Reed Army Institute of Research.

Bowman, J. (1967). *Recent experiences of combat psychiatry in Vietnam*. Unpublished manuscript. Division of Neuropsychiatry, Walter Reed Army Institute of Research, Washington, D.C.

Cardwell, T. A. (1985). Airland battle revisited. *Military Review*, *65* (9), 4–13.

Crocq, L., Crocq, M. A., Barrois, C., Belenky, G. L., and Jones, F. D. (1985). Low-intensity psychiatric casualties. In P. Pichot, P. Berner, R. Wolf, and K. Thau (eds.), *Psychiatry: the state of the art, Vol. 6*. New York: Plenum Press, pp. 545–550.

Dick, C. J. (1985a). Soviet operational concepts: part I. *Military Review*, *65* (9), 29–45.

Dick, C. J. (1985b). Soviet operational concepts: part II. *Military Review*, *65* (10), 4–19.

Drayer, C. S., and Glass, A. J. (1973). Introduction. In A. J. Glass (ed.), *Neuropsychiatry in World War II: Vol. 2. Overseas theaters*. Washington, D.C.: U.S. Government Printing Office, pp. 1–23.

El Sudany, M. G. (1982). Personal communication.

Gay, M. P. (1985). Soviet and U.S. operational styles of war. *Military Review*, *65* (9), 48–53.

Glass, A. J., Drayer, C. S., Cameron, D. C., and Woodward, W. D. (1954). Psychological first aid in community disasters. *Journal of the American Medical Association*, *156*, 36–41.

Glass, A. J. (1956). Psychotherapy in the combat zone. *American Journal of Psychiatry*, *110*(10).

Glass, A. J. (1957). Observations upon the epidemiology of mental illness in troops during warfare. Paper presented at the Symposium on Social Psychiatry, Walter Reed Army Institute of Research, WRAMC, Washington, D.C.

Glass, A. J. (1973). Lessons learned. In A. J. Glass (ed.). *Medical Depart-*

ment, *United States Army, Neuropsychiatry in World War II*: Vol. 2; Overseas theaters. Washington, D.C.: U.S. Government Printing Office, pp. 991–992.
Glass, A. J. (n.d.). *U.S. Army psychiatry in the Korean War era*, Chapter I: Army psychiatry before the Korean War era. (Unpublished manuscript). Department of Military Psychiatry, Walter Reed Army Institute of Research, Washington, D.C.
Griffith, S. B. (1963). *Sun Tzu: The Art of War*. New York: Oxford University Press, pp. 150–168.
Jones, F. D. (1967). Experiences of a division psychiatrist in Vietnam. *Military Medicine*, *132*(12), 1003–1008.
Jones, F. D. (1977). *Reactions to stress: combat versus combat-support psychiatric casualties*. Paper presented at VI World Congress of Psychiatry, Honolulu.
Jones, F. D. (1984a). *Psychiatric lessons of low-intensity wars*. Paper presented at World Psychiatric Association Regional Symposium, Helsinki, Finland. Also in press *Annales Medicine Militaris Fenniae*.
Jones, F. D. (1984b). *Challenges to combat psychiatry posed by the threat of nuclear warfare*. Paper presented at Army Medical Department Division and Combat Psychiatry Conference, Fort Bragg, N.C.
Jones, F. D. (1985a). Lessons of war for psychiatry. In P. Pichot, P. Berner, R. Wolf, and K. Thau (eds.), *Psychiatry: the state of the art, Vol. 6*. New York: Plenum Press, pp. 515–519.
Jones, F. D. (1985b). Sanctioned use of drugs in combat. In P. Pichot, P. Berner, R. Wolf, and K. Thau (eds.), *Psychiatry: the state of the art, Vol. 6*. New York: Plenum Press, pp. 489–494.
Jones, F. D., and Johnson, A. W. (1975). Medical and psychiatric treatment policy and practice in Vietnam. *Journal of Social Issues*, *31*(4), 49–65.
Keegan, J. (1976). *The face of battle*. New York: Viking Press.
Laughlin, H. P. (1967). *The neuroses*. Washington, D.C.: Butterworths, pp. 909–911.
Mansour, F. (1982). Manifestations of maladjustment to military service in Egypt after prolonged stress. *International Review of the Army, Navy, and Air Forces Medical Services*, *55*, 291–294.
Marlowe, D. H. (1985). Personal communication.
Mattila, M. J., Aranko, K., and Seppola, T. (1982). Acute effects of buspirone and alcohol on psychomotor skills. *Journal of Clinical Psychiatry*, *43*(12), 56–61.
Mohajer, M., and Mottaghi, Y. (1985). *Psychiatric war casualties in Iran*. Paper presented at American Psychiatric Association Annual Meeting, Dallas.

Moskowitz, H., and Smiley, A. (1982). Effects of chronically administered buspirone and diazepam on driving-related skills performance. *Journal of Clinical Psychiatry*, 43(12), 45–55.

Newton, R. E. (1983). Personal communication.

Paul, S. M. (1982). *Interactions of antidepressants and anxiolytics with neurotransmitter receptors: clinical implications*. Paper presented at Army Medical Department Military Psychiatry Conference, Uniformed Services University of the Health Sciences, Bethesda, Md.

Ranson, S. W. (1949). The normal battle reaction: its relation to the pathologic battle reaction. *Bulletin of the U.S. Army Medical Department, U.S. Armed Forces Medical Journal*, supplement entitled *Combat Psychiatry*, F. R. Hanson (ed.). Washington, D.C.: U.S. Government Printing Office, pp. 3–11.

Rosen, G. (1975). Nostalgia: a "forgotten" psychological disorder. *Psychological Medicine*, 5, 340–354.

Salmon, T. W. (1917). *The care and treatment of mental war and neuroses ("shell shock") in the British Army*. New York: War Work Committee of the National Committee for Mental Hygiene, Inc.

Skolnick, P., and Paul, S. M. (1981). Benzodiazepine receptors in the central nervous system. *International Review of Neurobiology*, 23, 102–140.

Snervais, S. (1979). "Forward detachments" and the Soviet nuclear offensive. *Military Review*, 49(4), 66–71.

Stouffer, S. A., DeVinney, L. C., Star, S. A., and Williams, R. M. (1949). *The American soldier, Vol. 2*. Princeton, N.J.: Princeton University Press.

Swank, R. L., and Marchand, W. E. (1946). Combat neuroses: development of combat exhaustion. *Archives of Neurology and Psychiatry*, 55, 236–247.

Tyhurst, J. S. (1951). Individual reactions to community disaster: the natural history of psychiatric phenomena. *American Journal of Psychiatry*, 107(3), 764–769.

Weinstein, E. A., and Drayer, C. S. (1949). A dynamic approach to the problem of combat-induced anxiety. In F. R. Hanson (ed.), *Combat psychiatry* (Supplement of the *Bulletin of the U.S. Army Medical Department*). Washington, D.C.: U.S. Government Printing Office.

Bibliographic Essay

Until recently, the subject of military psychiatry has not been the focus of serious academic or even medical concern in most countries. This is rather odd inasmuch as in every major war in this century—World War I, World War II, Korea, Vietnam, and the Israeli wars of 1973 and 1982—the number of soldiers lost to the fighting for psychiatric reasons has been greater than the number of soldiers killed. Nonetheless, few of the major military powers seem to have spent much time and effort in systematically assembling or conducting research on the subject of military psychiatry. What information exists, with the exception of the United States, are bits and pieces of medical, military, and academic research which have yet to be assembled in order to produce a coherent whole. This situation was the main stimulus for putting together this book.

If any one country can be said to have attempted to satisfactorily chronicle its experience with psychiatric breakdown in battle it is the military establishment of the United States. After World war II, President Eisenhower became concerned with the problem of manpower loss that he had witnessed while Commander-in-Chief of Allied Forces in Europe. His administration funded a major research effort in the area of combat psychiatry undertaken by a staff of researchers at Columbia University. The result was the first truly comprehensive treatment of the problem from the American perspective with the publication of Eli Ginzberg's, *The Lost Divisions* (New York: Columbia University Press, 1959). Much additional information on morale, cohesion, leadership, and the psychiatric condition of American troops in World War II can be found in S. A. Stouffer et al., *The American Soldier* (5 Vols.) (Princeton, N.J.: Princeton University Press, 1949). Two very valuable works that examine the structure and process of psychiatric breakdown in battle among American soldiers are J. W. Appel and G. W. Beebe, "Preventive Psychiatry: An Epidemiological Approach," *Journal of the American Medical Association* 131, (August 18, 1946) and A. J. Glass, "Observations Upon the Epidemiology of Mental Illness in Troops" (Washington, D.C.: U.S. Government Printing Office, 1954). An excellent source covering the experience of the American Army in World War I with psychiatric breakdown is found in Emanuel Miller, *Neurosis in War* (New York: MacMillan Co., 1942). This definitive and early work was totally ignored by the American military medical community during the interwar period. Had it remained in the military's consciousness, the military medical disasters of World War II may well have been prevented. It remains an excellent original source on the subject of combat psychiatry.

Among the best and most important works in the literature found anywhere, a work whose conclusions are applicable cross-culturally, is Roy Swank and Walter E. Marchand, "Combat Neuroses: Development of Combat Exhaustion," *Archives of Neurology and Psychiatry* 55, 1946. Swank and Marchand were the first to detail precisely the mental dynamics of psychiatric breakdown among combat soldiers. The work remains the best work yet published on the subject. A companion work, but one that is more historically oriented, is W. S. Mullens and A. J. Glass, eds., *Neuropsychiatry In World War II* Vol. 2 (Washington, D.C.: U.S. Government Printing Office, 1973).

The American experience with combat psychiatry in Vietnam has been only recently and incompletely chronicled. Among the best works on the subject are Franklin Jones and A. W. Johnson, "Medical and Psychiatric Treatment Policy and Practice in Vietnam," *Journal of Social Issues* 31, 1975 and T. Keane and J. Fairbanks, "Survey Analysis of Combat Related Stress Disorders in Vietnam Veterans," *American Journal of Psychiatry* 140, 1983. The definitive work is being written by Michael Camp, *Combat Psychiatry in Vietnam* (Westport, Conn.: Greenwood Press, forthcoming).

If the United States has more or less adequately recorded its experience with military psychiatry, the opposite extreme is represented by the availability of relevent literature on the subject dealing with the Soviet Union. To date only one book on the subject of Soviet military psychiatry has been published in the West. Thus, Richard A. Gabriel's, *Soviet Military Psychiatry* (Westport, Conn.: Greenwood Press, 1986), remains the definitive work. With regard to literature available in Soviet sources, this literature is scarce and unreliable. There are no sources worth noting that would add to the study of the subject by Russian-speaking scholars and military men.

The Germans have been very slow in producing any works on the subject relative to their own combat experience. The defeats suffered in two wars and the twisted racial and personality theories of the Nazi years made it all but impossible for German scholars and medical researchers to study the phenomenon of combat breakdown. Indeed, the chapter on German military psychiatry by Robert Schneider which appears in this book appears to be the first comprehensive attempt to produce an analysis of the problem among German troops in World War II. What exists as source literature is the usual bits and shards residing in unorganized archives, none of which offer a comprehensive overview of the subject. Nonetheless, among the most interesting of these shards is G. Elsaesser, "Erfahrung an 1400 Kriegsneurosen," *Psychiatrie der Gegenwart*, Volume 3 (Springer Verlag, 1961). Also of interest as it addresses the psychiatric impact of war on civilian populations in Germany is L. B. Kalinowsky, "War and Post-War Neuroses in Germany," *Medical Bulletin of the U.S. Army, Europe* (No. 3, March 1950). Among the better, if partial, sources available in English addressing the rates of psychiatric breakdown among German units in World War II is Martin Van Creveld, *Fighting Power: German and U.S. Army Performance, 1939–1945* (Westport, Conn.: Greenwood Press, 1983). Of general interest and background information is M. Simoneit, *Wehrpsychologie* (Berlin: Bernard and Graeffe, 1933). On the specific subject of war tremors, O. Wuth and C. Schneider, "Schuttel-Zitterer oder Kriegsneurotiker" (Berlin: April 4, 1942) can be found in the Militaerarchiv in Freiburg.

The Israelis are relative latecomers to the field of military psychiatry. Until the Yom Kipper War in 1973, they had experienced no significant degree of psychiatric breakdown among their soldiers. Accordingly, the subject commanded little attention from military medical personnel. In 1973, however, the problem emerged with a vengeance. In the 1973 war almost one-third of Israeli casualties were psychiatric. The Israeli response was to send a study team to the United States to learn the American theory and practice of dealing with battle-shock casualties. By 1980, once the data from the 1973 war were declassified, the Israelis began to produce any number of works of their own on the subject.

Most of the significant research emerged all at once and was published by the same source at the Third International Conference on Psychological Stress held in Tel Aviv in 1983. There exists as yet no complete and comprehensive work on the IDF's experience with combat shock, with the exception of Belenky's work which appears in this book.

Among the more interesting works produced by the Israelis is the work of Reuven Gal, "Characteristics of Heroism," published by the Conference in 1983. The work examines the background of 350 Israeli medal of honor winners in an attempt to locate those variables associated with heroism. But there are no significant variables associated with either heroism or cowardice. Published by the same source are M. Steiner and M. Neumann, "Traumatic Neurosis and Social Support in Yom Kippur War Returnees," which is a good source on how the Israelis deal with long-term psychiatric casualties. E. Kalay, "The Commander in Stress Situations in IDF Combat Units During the 'Peace for Galilee' Campaign," is typical of Israeli writings on the subject insofar as its reflects the Israeli belief that psychiatric casualties can be reduced if units retain strong social cohesion and trusted leadership.

As this essay makes painfully clear, there is a scarcity of source material on the subject of combat psychiatry in most countries. In this book, therefore, we have attempted to remedy some of this lack by presenting in a single source a number of complete and comprehensive works on the state of combat psychiatry in each of the major military powers. It is hoped that each military establishment will continue to produce additional studies as their own war experiences seem to merit. For the time being, however, this volume offers a detailed overview for the researcher wishing to avoid the disorganized literature which exists in each of the four countries studied.

Index

abasia, 115
abreaction, 152
Advanced Medical Battalion (AMB), 156, 159, 162, 164
aeroasthenia, 40
affective battle reactions, 111
affective flattening, 42
aloe, 89
ambulatory therapy, 165
American Expeditionary Force (AEF), 30, 32, 33, 183
American psychiatric losses in WW II, 2
Aminazine, 112, 113
Amitriptylene, 112
AMB, 156, 159, 162, 164
Ampriptylene, 112
anti-anxiety agents, 199
antipsychotics, 199
Arab-Israeli War of 1973, 2, 7, 12, 148, 153, 155, 171, 175, 177, 187, 195

armored personnel carrier, 95
army level hospitals, 81, 88, 96
astasia, 115
Australian forces, 14
autogenic training, 105
autonomic nervous system, 114
auto-suggestion, 105
AWOL, 10, 38, 133, 134

barbiturates, 199
battlefield paralysis, 191
Battle of the Bulge, 35
big psychiatry, 78
biological psychiatry, 77
biological shock, 104
Blitzkrieg, 127
Boer War, 67
brain shock, 83
Brickenstein, Rudolf, 126
bromides, 89, 199
buddy aid, 137, 140

INDEX

Bundeswher, 126
buspirone, 200

calcium chloride, 89, 113
cannabis, 199
Cannae, 6
cardiac bromide, 106
catatonia, 41
CFRU, 167
character disorder, 51, 53
character pathology, 168
Chlophophysine, 113
Chloprotixine, 112
Chloryl hydrate, 88, 106, 199
chronology of breakdown, 197
circular No. 293, 35
circular No. 370, 35
combat exhaustion, 48
combat fatigue, 10, 40, 41, 44, 52
Combat Fitness Retraining Unit, 166
combat reaction, 8, 10, 119, 149
combat zone fatigue, 50
commissariats, 72
commotion, 5, 182
conversion psychosis, 194
conversion reaction, 43
covert psychiatric casualties, 38
curative psychiatric tests, 86

Defense Intelligence Agency, 94
delayed battle shock, 149, 150, 165
delirium tremens, 122, 125
DEROS, 8, 18, 54
Dimedrol, 113
disorders of loneliness, 53, 182
disturbances of grasp, 42
drugs, major, in Soviet psychiatry, 104
DSM-III, 55
dull-wittedness, 92

Eleuterococus, 106
Elinium, 114, 115

Emisile, 114
emotional turmoil, 162
Encyclopedia of Military History, 71
Ensen shock treatment, 133
European Theater of Operations (ETO), 13
evacuation syndrome, 68, 198
exhaustion center stage, 42, 47
exogenic symptomatic psychosis, 115
expectancy, 79, 122, 132, 140, 184
explosion blow casualties, 183

failure to adapt, 72, 91
feldsher, 68, 69, 80, 81, 82, 97, 100
flying fatigue, 40
folk medicines, 71, 88
forward psychiatry, 129
forward treatment, 31, 154, 155, 162, 164, 176, 183
442 Regimental Combat Team, 13
fragging, 53
Freud, Sigmund, 123, 124
Freudian psychodynamics, 182
front psychiatry, 133
functional adjustment, 76

GABA, 115
ginseng, 89, 106
Glantz, Robert, 72, 74
Glass, A.J. 16
glucanated calcium, 113
goldroot, 89
group dynamics, 44

high intensity combat, 187, 190, 198
homesickness, 182
hyperstenic, 114
hypochondriasis, 123
hypostenic, 114
hysteria, 115, 123
hysterical neurosis, 115, 137

INDEX

ICD-9, 91, 106
Ilenium, 112
imbecillia, 73, 92
immaturity reactions, 51
immediacy, 79, 122, 140
Institute of Forensic Psychiatry, 91, 92
Israeli Defense Force (IDF), 156, 171; mental health clinic, 158, 159; mental health department, 159

Kaufmann method, 84, 132
killed in action, WW II, American Army, 10, 12
Kirov Military Medical Academy, 110
Kraepelin, Emile, 28
kriegsneurose, 126, 134
kriegsschuettler, 131
kriegszitterer, 137

Leningrad Military District Hospital, 99
leonuria, 106
Levopromozene, 112, 113
leuzeue, 106
low intensity conflict, 185, 188, 189
L-pheylalanine, 199
L-tyrosine, 199

mandarin root, 89
manic depressive psychosis, 122
Marchand, W.E., 10
Marshall, S.L.A., 45
mass panic, 27
Meggido, 6
Melipramine, 112
Meprobamate, 114
microbleeding, 5, 83, 183
Minnesota Multiphasic Personality Inventory (MMPI), 167
mixed syndromes, 158

molecular derangement, 182
mutism, 115

National Committee for Mental Hygiene, 29, 30
natrium bromide, 89
neurasthenia, 70, 89, 114, 182
neurotransmitters, 199
Nisei, 13
nostalgia, 181, 182

old sergeants syndrome, 39, 42, 49
oligaphrenia, 92
operational fatigue, 40
operational mobile group, 190

PLO, 156
pantacrene, 106
paresis, 122
penatine, 109
People's Commissariat of Public Health, 106
Perheneazine, 112
pharmacological era of psychiatry, 104
Phenamine, 109
Phenaput, 110
Phenazapen, 112
Phenazecom, 114
Phenazepam, 112
Phynazepam, 115
phobia, 173
Political Academy, 102
post-traumatic stress disorder (PTSD), 55
powdered reindeer horn, 89
primary groups, 22
principle of expectancy, 87, 90
principle of immediacy, 90
proximity, 68, 79, 90, 122, 140, 183
psychiatric assistants, 100
psychiatric screening, 34

psychogenic disturbances, 140
psychomotor disturbances, 121
psychosomatic casualties, 201
Pyrazdol, 112

reactive delirious psychosis, 112-13
reactive states, 110
Reichenau, General von, 128
replacement batallion, 94
replacement depots, 94, 95
revolution in psychopharmacology, 90
rules for psychoneurosis wards, 32
Russian casualties, WW II, 71
Russian Red Cross Society, 68
Russo-Japanese War, 25, 67, 68, 69, 70, 71, 79

St. Elizabeth's Hospital, 28
Salmon, Thomas, 30, 183
screening conscripts, 90
search and avoid, 53
secondary gain, 69, 70, 131
second-echelon psychiatric care, 165
self help for the soldier, 198
self-inflicted wounds, 121, 133
shallow depression, 112
shell shock, 29, 41, 122, 183
short timers syndrome, 49, 158, 175
Siduzin, 112
Sindophine, 114
situational clusters, 154
small psychiatry, 78, 113
social support, 44
socio-rehabilitative theories, 103
sodium amytal, 46
sodium bromide, 89
somatic complaints, 121
Sovgexin, 114
Spiegel, Herbert, 15
Spivak, L.I., 110

stable personality, 151
startle reaction, 41
Sun Tzu, 181
supportive psychotherapy, 152
surdomutism, 79, 84, 194
Swank, R.L., 10, 197
Swiss disease, 181
Syndocarb, 109, 114

technical fixes, 24
theories of second sort, 56
ticket-in, 164
ticket-out, 79, 83, 88, 164
Tisercin, 112
torpillage, 124
transient anxiety reaction, 119
transitional personality, 151
Trapazine, 114
traumatic encephalopathy, 83
Triftazin, 112
Trioxizine, 110, 114
Trisedil, 112
twilight states, 115

udar, 76
unsuitability, 91

Valadium, 89
valeriana, 106
vegeostabilizers, 114
Vietnam, 14

war neurosis, 32, 40, 135
Waterloo, 6
weak will, 125
Wehrmacht, 120
work batallion, 135
wounded in action (WIA), 10, 148

Yom Kippur War, 14

Contributors

GREGORY LUCAS BELENKY, M.D., is Chief of the Department of Behavioral Biology of the Walter Reed Army Institute of Research and Associate Professor of Psychiatry at the Uniformed Services University of the Health Sciences. He holds the rank of Lieutenant Colonel in the U.S. Army.

RICHARD A. GABRIEL is Professor of Politics at St. Anselm College. He is the author of eighteen books and scores of articles on military subjects and has written the first book on Soviet military psychiatry ever published in the West.

LAWRENCE INGRAHAM serves as a health services research psychologist at the Walter Reed Army Institute of Research. He has a doctorate in social psychology and holds the rank of Lieutenant Colonel in the U.S. Army.

FRANKLIN D. JONES, M.D., is the Associate Director for Combat Stress, Neuropsychiatry Division, of the Walter Reed Army Institute of Research and a Professor at the Georgetown University Medical School and the Uniformed University of the Health Sciences. He holds the rank of Colonel in the U.S. Army.

FREDERICK MANNING has a doctorate in experimental psychology from Harvard and is the Deputy Director of the Division of Neuropsychiatry at the Walter Reed Army Institute of Research. He is a Lieutenant Colonel in the U.S. Army.

DAVID MARLOWE is Chairman of the Department of Military Psychiatry at the Walter Reed Army Institute of Research in Washington, D.C. and holds a Ph.D. from Harvard University.

ROBERT SCHNEIDER is the former Chief of the Department of Neuropsychiatry at the Armed Forces Institute of Medicine in Bangkok and Commander of the U.S. Army Medical Research Unit, Europe. He holds a Ph.D. and is a Lieutenant Colonel in the U.S. Army assigned as a research psychologist at the Walter Reed Army Institute of Research in Washington.

**Recent Titles in
Contributions in Military Studies**

The Tainted War: Culture and Identity in Vietnam War Narratives
Lloyd B. Lewis

Shaping a Maritime Empire: The Commercial and Diplomatic Role of the American Navy, 1829–1861
John H. Schroeder

The American Occupation of Austria: Planning and Early Years
Donald R. Whitnah and Edgar L. Erickson

Crusade in Nuremberg: Military Occupation, 1945–1949
Boyd L. Dastrup

The Dogma of the Battle of Annihilation: The Theories of Clausewitz and Schlieffen and Their Impact on the German Conduct of Two World Wars
Jehuda L. Wallach

Jailed for Peace: The History of American Draft Law Violators, 1658–1985
Stephen M. Kohn

Against All Enemies: Interpretations of American Military History from Colonial Times to the Present
Kenneth J. Hagan and William R. Roberts

Citizen Sailors in a Changing Society: Policy Issues for Manning the United States Naval Reserve
Louis A. Zurcher, Milton L. Boykin, and Hardy L. Merritt, editors

Strategic Nuclear War: What the Superpowers Target and Why
William C. Martel and Paul L. Savage

Soviet Military Psychiatry: The Theory and Practice of Coping with Battle Stress
Richard A. Gabriel

A Portrait of the Israeli Soldier
Reuven Gal

The Other Price of Hitler's War: German Military and Civilian Losses Resulting from World War II
Martin K. Sorge

The New Battlefield: The United States and Unconventional Conflicts
Sam C. Sarkesian